THE
ROYAL MARINES
CIRCUIT
TRAINING

The All-round Commando Fitness Programme

Robin Eggar & Dieter Loraine

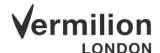

Vermilion
LONDON

Once again with all my love to Jacqui, Jordan and Rowan
ROBIN EGGAR

To Denise, my wife, and my sons, Jordan and Dieter, for putting up with me and my various exploits throughout our marriage
DIETER LORAINE

First published in the United Kingdom in 1996 by Vermilion, an imprint of Ebury Press, Random House,
20 Vauxhall Bridge Road, London SW1V 2SA

Random House Australia (Pty) Limited
20 Alfred Street, Milsons Point, Sydney
New South Wales 2061, Australia

Random House New Zealand Limited
18 Poland Road, Glenfield
Auckland 10, New Zealand

Random House South Africa (Pty) Limited
Endulini, 5A Jubilee Rd, Parktown 2193, South Africa

Random House Group Limited Reg. No. 954009

www.randomhouse.co.uk

ISBN: 0091888700

Editors: Jan Bowmer and Nicky Thompson
Designed from disk by Roger Walker
Photographs: Jon Stewart

Printed and bound in Great Britain by
Scotprint, Haddington, East Lothian

Papers used by Ebury Press are natural recyclable products made from wood grown in sustainable forests.

ACKNOWLEDGMENTS

Technical advisors:
Sergeant Paul Gellender who provided invaluable information on diet and remedial circuits.
Corporal Paul 'Jumper' Collin who designed several sports specific circuits.

Trainers:
Corporal Al Stacey
Warrant Officer Chris Butler

This book would not have been possible without the tremendous experience and vital cooperation of the Physical Training Branch of the Royal Marines. Special thanks to: Captain John Glaze and Colour Sergeant Paul Rees of the Royal Marines Public Relations Department; Brigadier Roger Dillon and Warrant Officer Nigel Devenish at Lympstone Commando, Training Centre. Also, thanks to Major General Andrew Keeling for writing the Foreword – good luck with the St Dunstan's Appeal.

Robin Eggar would like to thank Nike, Rockport and Tunturi for making and providing kit that is comfortable and actually lasts; his civilian trainer George Ellis for both keeping him up to par and loaning bits of kit for photographs, and Simon Costain who taught him how to like (if not yet love) his feet.

Thanks are also due to our agent Julian 'the Terrier' Alexander, Jon Stewart who has now become very accomplished at photographing Marine PTIs in various stages of undress, and Fiona MacIntyre, Jan Bowmer and Nicky Thompson for translating exercises, words and scrawled diagrams into this book.

WARNING: If you have a medical condition or are pregnant, you should not under any circumstances follow the programme in this book without first consulting your doctor. All guidelines and warnings should be read carefully and the authors and publishers cannot accept responsibility for injuries or damage arising out of a failure to comply with the same.

Contents

Foreword

Royal Marines are sea-soldiers. They are part of the Royal Navy but they exist to fight on land. They therefore need to know how to retain their fitness while they are cooped up on their ships in confined spaces, often for quite long periods. They are also all Commandos, and this means that they have to be ready at all times to go, at very short notice, to any part of the world to resolve a crisis. Commandos are not supermen – they are ordinary people – but they are specifically trained to handle crises in arduous and inhospitable terrain where they are likely to be severely tested physically.

In my short 33 years as a Royal Marine I was involved in emergency situations in the jungles of Borneo, in the Radfan mountains and the deserts of southern Arabia, in the baking heat of the mid-summer Cyprus sun, in the South Atlantic during the Falklands War, and in the extremely inhospitable Zagros mountains of North Iraq at the end of the Gulf War (when the Commando Brigade helped to resettle thousands of Kurdish refugees). I also spent years training in the Norwegian Arctic where low temperatures, deep snow and high mountains make huge demands on the human body and brain.

In my early twenties, I qualified as a Royal Marines Physical Training Officer, and became one of the very few officers to join the Physical Training Branch. I ran all PT and sport at the Royal Navy's College in Dartmouth, and subsequently was responsible for training all Royal Marines Physical Training Instructors. I played squash and hockey at inter-service and county level and have always played a lot of various sports.

But, apart from the sheer fun of keeping fit and competing, I realised early on in my adult life that being physically fit has a tremendous spin-off on your capacity to think and to concentrate, particularly when under pressure. The motto of the Royal Marines Physical Training Branch is *mens sana in corpore sano* (a healthy mind in a healthy body). I have found this to be a very appropriate motto for people who regularly face challenges of any sort: physical challenges, mental challenges or both. There is absolutely no doubt that your brain will work better and for longer if your body is in good shape.

Commandos go through a very tough training course when they first join the Royal Marines and they are then required to keep themselves fit throughout the rest of their service. Becoming really fit and strong, with deep reserves of stamina, builds tremendous confidence – and it is this inner confidence in self and team which is a real winner in any difficult situation. All over the world I have seen young Commandos take arduous conditions in their stride with amazing cheerfulness and confidence. Most of this impressive ability to cope cheerfully with harsh weather, inhospitable terrain, spartan living conditions, to say nothing of a determined enemy, is due to the confidence that comes with being in peak physical condition.

I recently saw a very short TV interview with a young Royal Marine in Bosnia. He was about 19 years old, of slight build and, except for the uniform and the situation, he looked a little like a displaced choirboy. He was standing in the snow and had an enormous load on his back. The interviewer, with a slightly cynical sneer to his voice, asked the Marine 'And how far are you going to carry all that?', to which the young man replied in a matter-of-fact way 'As far as I'm told to'. That said it all, for this young man had gained sufficient confidence from his Commando training to know that he could do anything that was required of him. And the inner strength that this confidence gives is a winner in any situation: on the battlefield, in the boardroom, or even when trying to fight your way out of a bunker on the golf course.

Being physically fit also makes you feel good. I am now the wrong side of 50, but I felt good when my doctor told me the other day that I have the blood pressure of a teenager. I know that my apparently healthy state owes much to the fact that I have always watched my diet and weight, and have done my best to maintain a good level of fitness.

And why have I done this? Partly because as a Royal Marine I needed to, but equally as much it is because it makes me feel good. It's also because I know that if I am in good physical shape there is more of a chance that my mind will shape up to any challenge or crisis which I face, and of my body not letting me down when I need it to continue for that extra mile.

This book will help you get in shape, and stay in shape for life. It isn't a book for budding supermen: it won't give you huge muscles. It will, however, guide you through a programme of progressive physical exercises which, combined with a healthy regard for diet, rest, alcohol and nicotine, will give you *mens sana in corpore sano*. Both Robin Eggar and Dieter Loraine have good reason (as I do) to know that the recipe works. I hope you enjoy making it work too.

MAJOR GENERAL ANDREW KEELING CH, CBE

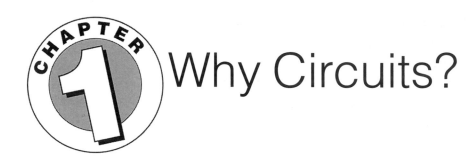

Why Circuits?

In 1982 Dieter Loraine was serving with 45 Commando when they were sent to the Falklands. 'Once we were on board our troop ships, we embarked on a strict regime of yomping (carrying over 100 lb of equipment each) and circuit training,' he recalls, 'and without this we would not have been able to do the famous 50-mile yomp to Port Stanley. Circuits build stamina and endurance, and being fit increased our ability to concentrate for longer periods and act faster under pressure. The ultimate pressure is the threat of *death* at any moment. I can honestly say that, at the time, the Royal Marines were the fittest soldiers in the world – bred on a diet of daily circuit training.

'On returning from the campaign we were on the *Canberra*. It was too crowded for us to run or have military training on board but every vacant space from the cabins to the holds was transformed into a troop circuit training den. Even when relaxing and recovering from war the Marines still circuit trained – voluntarily.' Circuit training works for the Royal Marines, in peace and in war. But what relevance does it have for civilians?

In 1994 Robin Eggar wrote an article for *Esquire* magazine in which he tried to answer a seemingly impossible question – 'Who is Britain's fittest sportsman?' Are sprinters fitter than cyclists? Do swimmers have better endurance than squash players? Such things are never definitive but using a series of seven tests, designed by the Human Performance Centre at Lilleshall to demonstrate all-round fitness, the magazine tested sportsmen, athletes, dancers and a Royal Marines Physical Training Instructor.

Overall Colin Jackson, the 110 metre hurdler, came first but what was fascinating was how certain professional sport disciplines can lead to an unbalanced body. In other words, in certain areas they are not as fit as they seem. For example, Olympic gold medal cyclist Chris Boardman has incredibly powerful legs, phenomenal lung capacity and boundless stamina. Yet his upper body appears almost translucent, with no fat and no muscle definition. He has very little upper body strength. This doesn't matter to Boardman because every extra pound he weighs is another pound to drag over the Alps on the Tour de France. Similarly, Matthew Yates, an 800 and 1500 metre specialist, has phenomenal endurance yet he cannot touch his toes – but then he has no need to. Neither Boardman nor Yates need all-round ability.

Although Jackson won, the best all-round performances came from champions in sports not exactly overflowing with glamour and big bucks. Both gymnast Neil Thomas and Ray Stevens, a judo silver medalist at the Barcelona Olympics, require an all-round fitness – they need both aerobic and anaerobic capabilities. Other than sports specific training, the core of both of their training schedules was doing circuits, which they used to boost their all-round fitness to a higher peak.

Perhaps surprisingly, perhaps not, the most impressive all-round performance came from Ross Barbour, the Royal Marines PTI and a downhill skier for the Navy. In all seven tests Ross never finished below fifth place, an incredible achievement for an amateur competing against some of the nation's best athletes. Unlike the training schedules followed by Jackson, Barbour's training was all done in Marine gymnasiums, either 'beasting' (the affectionate term for 'training') recruits, or driving himself through an intensive set of circuits.

Circuits also worked for Robin Eggar who did the tests and is not ashamed of his performance. 'For the record I came last overall (but last in only three of the seven tests). Not only was I the oldest by a decade, I was also the only real amateur. My training schedule had consisted of running twice a week and a thrice weekly circuit adapted from my first exercise book, *Royal Marines Total Fitness*. The firmest conclusion I came to after we finished was not who was the fittest sportsman, but what was the best way to get fit: old-fashioned no-frills circuit training.'

But are circuits so old fashioned? Today there are machines for everything. Except most don't really work, and those that do carry out the mechanical and physical tasks for which they were designed are no fun. Do you really want to spend a fortune going down the gym, to be baffled by banks of hi-tech machinery, to work out on a lump of metal that tells you how many calories you might have burned off in a 20-minute session? Why stay in a sweaty room and run three miles on an ergonomically designed treadmill when you can spin round the local park, catch some fresh air and often some pretty interesting sights.

Fitness is not just about physical jerks; it involves both mind and body. At times it hurts like hell but in the final analysis we take exercise because we enjoy it. Unnecessary complications detract from that enjoyment. Efficient exercise needs to be simple. Circuits are simple and effective.

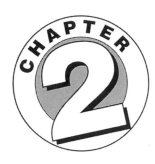

How to Use This Book

The programme in this book is designed to take a 'fat civvy' (which is how the Marines refer to all new recruits – they become Nods when they have passed their Initial Military Fitness tests) to a level of physical fitness where he can pass a formidable physical test. To get the major benefits:

1 Read Chapters 1 and 3. They explain the physical benefits of circuit training and how important it is to take a Whole Body Approach (WBA). Follow our recommendations on diet (Chapter 5).
2 Answer the questionnaires in Chapter 4. If you are in any doubt consult a doctor before starting the Nod Circuit Programme (Chapter 8).
3 Make sure you have all the basic kit you require (see opposite).
4 DO NOT SKIP Chapter 6 on Warming Up, Cooling Down and Stretching – this is an *essential* part of the training and is aimed to increase your flexibility and prevent injuries.
5 Even if you are already tolerably fit, follow the programme from Week 1.
6 Keep up the maintenance programme in Chapter 9.
7 If you are a sports enthusiast, look at the Sports Specific Circuits (Chapter 10) after you have completed the Nod Circuit Programme.
8 If you are up to it, tackle the SBS Challenge (Chapter 11).
9 Consult the Appendices for extra information on foot care, tips on avoiding injury and remedial advice.
10 Refer to the Exercise Index to find all the individual circuit exercises used in the book, especially if you want to design your own circuit.

What Kit Do You Need?

Not a lot! Don't run out and spend a fortune on all the latest gadgets, the coolest running shoes, designer sportswear and machines that monitor your pulse rate. Wearing a running vest with a go-faster stripe doesn't make you go quicker, just as wearing the smartest ski suits doesn't mean you can suddenly ski a black run. You will already have most of what you need in the way of T-shirts, shorts and sweat pants. Exercise in what makes you feel comfortable, not in what Linford Christie wears when he's winning medals.

BASIC ESSENTIALS

Trainers

Trainers are the one item that you should not stint on. Do **not** wear running shoes during circuit training. Wear cross trainers, aerobic shoes with a low-cut heel, tennis or squash shoes – anything that provides a bit of uppers support when you turn and jump. For further advice see page 132.

Training clothes

Basics should include at least two sets of the following: Vest/T-shirt, shorts, sports socks (Thor-Lo are highly recommended), one track suit (shell suits are a definite no-no and sweat bottoms get heavy when wet so be aware of this when exercising outside). If you intend to exercise outside on dark winter mornings or evenings you should also have a woolly hat, gloves, and a fluorescent vest and/or reflective ankle bands for running. Change your kit after each session; keep it clean and dry to avoid picking up any infections or smelling.

Sports watch

Beg, borrow or buy one. We recommend sports watches by Timex and Casio that have stop watch, lap and beep functions all built in.

Water

Wherever you are exercising make sure that you have water ready to hand. If you are doing circuits inside then have a jug and glass standing by. If you're outside take a full 1.5 litre bottle (bike bottles are cheap and unbreakable). Drink constantly.

Access to a bicycle

To broaden your horizons during those Active Rest days, you really need a bike. A static exercise bike will do initially but it is a cop-out as it does not allow for changes in terrain, climatic conditions and so forth. It also gets boring not going anywhere. Most gyms/health clubs now have sophisticated computer-programmed bikes, so explain to the assistant what you want to do. Mountain bikes with their wider tyres and tougher frames are generally better for big city potholes than racing bikes – but they are heavier to ride. If you are going to cycle exclusively on town roads, consider using the new hybrid bikes, which combine mountain-bike technology in a lighter-weight frame.

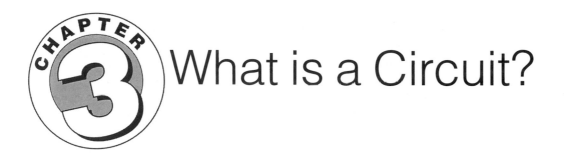

CHAPTER 3

What is a Circuit?

The Royal Marines Physical Training Branch states that:

> **'The aim of circuit training is the progressive development of the muscular and circulo-respiratory system. Circuit training achieves all-round fitness.'**

The circuit is certainly at the very core of all physical exercise training and of *any* physical discipline – whether it be football or mountaineering – that requires a high level of fitness. It may not be called a 'circuit' but that is what it is. Different sports may all require different levels of fitness and strength in different areas of the body but it is important to keep a balance and tone other areas of the body. The only efficient way to tone yourself is to do repetitive exercises on specific muscle groups – circuits. These are what the Royal Marines have been doing for years.

What is Physical Fitness?

Fitness means different things to different people. When we say someone looks fit we are usually referring to an immediate surface impression, a condition of apparent wellbeing, and of looking good, all of which are often confused with being healthy. Being physically fit does not mean being healthy.

We need to differentiate between total and physical fitness. Total fitness is the ability to meet the demands of the environment, with a little left in reserve for emergencies. It includes physical, mental, emotional, social, medical and nutritional fitness. If you have the first – physical fitness – you establish a fertile soil in which the others can take root.

Physical fitness requires the heart, blood vessels, lungs and muscles to function at optimum efficiency, enabling an individual to be able to indulge in daily tasks, sport and recreation with a physical and mental enthusiasm that makes them all the more pleasurable. Optimum physical fitness makes possible a lifestyle that the unfit cannot enjoy unless they too wish to develop and maintain a similar level of physical fitness. It requires dedication, vigorous effort and does not come easy.

There are five components to physical fitness:

1 **Cardiovascular fitness** (sometimes referred to as endurance, stamina or aerobic power). Cardiovascular fitness means you have a fit heart and circulatory system. Aerobic activities improve the efficiency and capacity of the heart and lungs in transporting oxygen to active muscles.

2 **Muscular strength** Strength is the ability of a muscle or group of muscles to exert maximum force to overcome a resistance. By progressively increasing the amount of resistance a muscle must overcome, it will be trained to work more efficiently. In weight training a person will become stronger by increasing either the weight lifted or the number of times that the weight is lifted. All movement and sports require muscular strength. Poor muscular strength often leads to skeletal muscular strains and pulls.

3 **Muscular endurance** The ability of a muscle or group of muscles to exert force to overcome resistance and to work continuously over an extended period of time. To achieve endurance in weight training light weights are used and the number of reps significantly increased.

4 **Flexibility** The ability to use either muscles and/or the skeletal joints throughout their full range of movement. Mobility is another term used to describe this component. However, mobility is more commonly used to refer to gentle rhythmic movements taken up to but not beyond the range of movement in the joint or muscle (eg neck and arm circling, cycling while lying on the back). Also called 'limbering' or 'loosening up', this is generally used as part of a warm-up to prepare the joints and muscles for exercise.

Flexibility exercises involve stretching the muscles and are directly aimed at extending the range of movement of a joint or muscle. The term 'stretching' has come to be accepted as describing these kind of exercises though technically the muscles are relaxing. Stretches must be performed statically and only after the body has been properly warmed up.

5 **Motor skills fitness** This refers to factors such as agility, balance, reaction time, coordination, and speed, and is sometimes also described as 'mental fitness'.

Why circuit training is an ideal form of fitness training

- It is flexible, adaptable, enjoyable, simple and progressive.
- Enables individuals or groups to take part.
- Individuals can work at their own pace.
- Can be adapted to suit all levels of ability.
- Can be adapted to all sports.
- Uses little or no equipment.
- Can be carried out in very confined spaces (ships, offices, front room etc).
- Offers variety in exercises.
- Boredom very rarely sets in if planned well.

If you are aiming to meet the demands of daily life – with that little bit in reserve – you must achieve a certain level of fitness in each of these five components. It is possible to have a high score in one and low in another. A weight-lifter will score very high on strength and flexibility but may lack cardiovascular fitness, while runners may score high on cardiovascular fitness but lack strength in the upper body.

Circuit training aims to develop and increase your fitness in all five components of physical fitness. If you embark on one specific training regime you will not increase general muscular strength and toning and you may overdevelop certain specific muscle areas. Circuit training exercises the whole body leading to a systematic whole body conditioning process. It is the most effective method of overall body conditioning and has the added benefit of cutting down on injuries to overused individual muscle groups that specific trainers, like runners, cyclists and swimmers, routinely receive.

The very nature, the essence of circuit training is that it helps to develop all-round fitness as opposed to fitness for a specific sport. Exercises that do relate to sport events can and are included in particular circuits. However the prime value of circuit training is the development of *general* fitness through exercising and developing the muscular and circulo-respiratory system (the heart and lungs to us civvies).

The different types of circuit

The Royal Marines Physical Training Instructors use four different types of circuit – they are neither harder nor easier than each other, just different. All are designed to enable them to train groups of 30 men at any one time – and keep an eye on them. The difficulty and challenge that each circuit offers is dependent on the amount and type of exercise in each circuit.

1 Timed Circuit

For a large group, parts of the gym are assigned as individual exercise stations. Individuals are given a set time to work at each of these. It should not be so long that the exerciser loses the ability to carry out the exercise properly and starts to cheat, but it should be long enough for everyone to 'get into the activity' and work progressively to the end of the time. 15-30 seconds is a good guide. There should be an adequate rest time after each exercise.

2 Individual Circuit

The procedure for this is explained in detail later. The Individual Circuit provides the Test you will be taking three times in the Nod Circuit Programme

(Chapter 8). In essence you are competing with yourself to do a set number of exercises within a specified Target Time.

3 Repetition Circuit (or Colour Circuit)

Imagine 12 different exercise stations. There is a board by each station detailing the exercise. On each board there will also be three numbers: 12 coloured in Blue, 10 in Yellow and 8 in Red. You are told to carry out three complete circuits using only the Yellow numbers, so each exercise you reach must be performed 10 times. Or the first circuit is Blue, the second Yellow, the third Red, as you start to flag.

If you are training a group with different fitness levels a colour circuit is particularly useful in allowing you to differentiate between abilities. Beginners do Red circuits only, those at intermediate level do Yellow only, while the advanced animals stick to Blue.

4 Running Circuit

This is a real beast and is done in a park or on a running track. You have a list of exercises which must be repeated three times, 12 repetitions on the first circuit, 10 on the second and 8 on the third. You set your watch to beep at one-minute intervals. When it beeps you stop, do the necessary reps, leap to your feet and jog on until the watch beeps again… and so on. The theory behind this is that the faster you do the reps the more time you have to recover before the next set – the idea being that you recover while running!

In this book we use variations on all four of the Marine circuits but as we expect most people to be training either alone or in pairs, they have been tailored to the individual. As you go through the Nod Circuit Programme, the format and content of the circuits change which adds variety and helps to prevent boredom.

The six circuit commandments

1 Warm up and down thoroughly.

2 Understand fully the exercises to be carried out prior to starting the circuit.

3 Exercise the whole body (injuries permitting). Take a Whole Body Approach (WBA).

4 Do not exercise any one muscle group consecutively (unless training specifically for a certain sport or activity).

5 Work to your own limits.

6 Carry out exercises properly – do not cheat on the full range of movement.

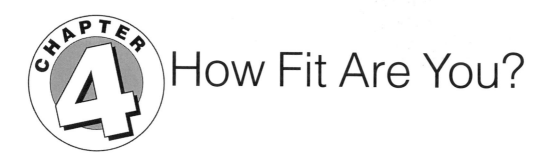

How Fit Are You?

Before he is selected as a recruit, every potential Marine has to go through a medical and various other tests to prove his suitability for the role he is undertaking. This chapter is designed to get you to ask and answer questions about your body and your approach to physical fitness, and keep a record of how your physical shape and fitness are improving.

Monitoring Pulse Rates

To help monitor your level of fitness, you need to know about four pulse rates. You can find your pulse either at the main artery on the side of your neck, just below the junction of the jaw, or on the flat side of your wrist in line with your thumb. Press with the first two fingers and count the number of beats. It is more accurate to take the pulse over a full minute though if rushed you can take it for 15 seconds and multiply by 4, or 10 seconds and multiply by 6.

1 **Resting pulse rate** When you wake up in the morning after a good night's sleep, take your rate for a minute. Do this for three days and take the average as your resting rate. In the future if the rate is over 10 beats per minute (bpm) higher than that average do not train during the day because you are too tired to do so.

2 **Working rate** Check what your rate is after a normal morning's activity. On average it should tend to be 10 bpm higher than the resting rate. If your rate has been too high on waking but has returned to normal during the day then you can consider training again.

3 **Maximum heart rate** Simply deduct your age in years from 220. This is your approximate Maximum Heart Rate (MHR) – the maximum amount your heart can beat in a minute. Above that you are pushing yourself too hard and depriving the blood of oxygen.

4 **Target heart rate zone** When exercising aerobically, you should aim to work out at between 60 and 80 per cent of your MHR. This is your target heart rate zone. However to begin with you should not work at levels above 75 per cent MHR. If you do not achieve this for more than 20 minutes at least three times a week you are not actually increasing your training capability.

General Questions

1 Physical measurements

Note down:

- Age _____
- Height _____
- Weight _____
- Measure the following and note the widest measurements:

  Stomach _____

  Thighs _____

  Chest _____

  Biceps _____

  Calves _____

- Do the fat test. Most gyms can do a proper test with callipers and charts but for a basic rule of thumb do the pinch test. Take a pinch of flesh between thumb and forefinger in the following four places:

  Biceps _____

  Triceps _____

  Beneath the shoulder blade _____

  One inch above and along from the hip bone _____

- Check your resting pulse rate (sit down and relax for 20 minutes then take your pulse or take it first thing in the morning – see opposite)

Keep a note of your weight, pinches and measurements for later on.

2 Lifestyle

- Do you drink, if so how much and how regularly?
- Do you smoke?
- Do you need a strong cup of coffee or a cigarette to get going in the morning?
- What is the basic constituent of your diet?
- Are you dieting or have you tried to diet in the past? How successful were you?
- Is your energy level less than it used to be?

continued

3 Exercise

- Do you exercise less than one hour a week?   ☐ Yes ☐ No
- Is your job one where you're seated all day?   ☐ Yes ☐ No
- Were you fitter:
  - ☐ 5 years ago?
  - ☐ 10 years ago?
  - ☐ Longer ago than you care to admit even to yourself?

4 Diet

- Do you eat fried food more than three times a week?   ☐ Yes ☐ No
- Do you eat red meat more than three times a week?   ☐ Yes ☐ No
- Is your diet moderate to high fat (do you cook in oil/fat/butter and eat cooked fat/skin on meat)?   ☐ Yes ☐ No
- Are you a meat eater?   ☐ Yes ☐ No
- Do you eat full-fat dairy products (full-fat milk, yogurt, cheese, butter) every day?   ☐ Yes ☐ No
- Do you eat less than five portions of either fresh fruit, salads and vegetables every day?   ☐ Yes ☐ No
- Do you eat biscuits, cakes, chocolate or sweets regularly?   ☐ Yes ☐ No
- Do you eat more than three eggs (yolk and white) a week?   ☐ Yes ☐ No
- Do you drink more than three units of alcohol a day?   ☐ Yes ☐ No
  (A unit is the equivalent of a small glass of wine; a pub measure of spirits; $1/2$ pint of ordinary beer, lager or cider; or $1/4$ pint of strong beer, lager or cider.)
- Do you eat pulses/ wholemeal bread less than three times a week?   ☐ Yes ☐ No

If you answered **Yes** to more than four of the diet questions you should consider making gradual changes to your diet by following our tips in Chapter 5.

5 Motivation

- Why do you want to get fit?
- Did you buy this book, or did someone give it to you?
- Will this book make you fit, or will you make yourself fit?

Think about your answers.

Pre-exercise medical questionnaire

You **must** answer **Yes** or **No** to the following questions:

1 Has your doctor ever said you have heart disease or any other cardiovascular problem? ☐ Yes ☐ No

2 Is there a history of heart disease in your family? ☐ Yes ☐ No

3 Has your doctor ever said you have high blood pressure? ☐ Yes ☐ No

4 Do you ever have pains in your heart and chest after undergoing minimal exertion? ☐ Yes ☐ No

5 Do you often get headaches, feel faint or dizzy? ☐ Yes ☐ No

6 Do you suffer from pain or limited movement in any joints or bones which have either been aggravated by exercise or might be made worse by it? ☐ Yes ☐ No

7 Are you taking drugs or medication, or recuperating from a recent illness or operation at the moment? ☐ Yes ☐ No

8 Do you have any other condition which might affect your ability to participate in exercise? ☐ Yes ☐ No

9 Are you over 35 and unaccustomed to physical exercise? ☐ Yes ☐ No

If you answered **Yes** to one or more questions consult your doctor **before** starting circuit training. Ask his or her advice as to whether you can undertake unrestricted physical training/activity on a gradually increasing basis. If your doctor suggests only restricted or supervised activities for an initial period discuss whether circuit training will fulfil these criteria.

If you answered **No** to all the questions you should feel reasonably assured that you are ready to begin.

However if you have a temporary illness, even as seemingly minor as a case of the snuffles, a cough or a slight sore throat, **postpone** starting the exercise programme until you are fully recovered. We want you to enjoy it and there is nothing worse than starting off when you feel like you've been run over by a truck. Circuit training may be tough but we want it to be fun.

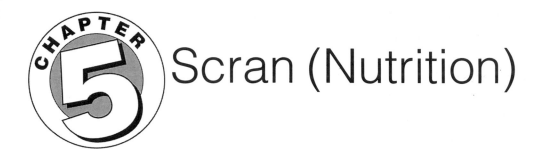

Scran (Nutrition)

Welcome to a chapter on the Royal Marines Total Dieting, Cooking for a Healthier, Happier Lifestyle. Only joking! But it's a misconception that real Marines don't diet or cook – they do if they want to achieve all-round physical fitness.

The chances are that, like the majority of the population, you are a few pounds overweight. You would love to shed that unwanted flab and maybe an inch or two off your tummy. The only way to lose fat is to consume fewer calories than your body uses – to eat less and burn off more. So the best way to lose fat is through a combination of diet and exercise. One way to do this, without endangering your health, is to select a different combination of foods that will supply your body with the balanced intake of nutrients it needs but in fewer calories. This is not as easy as simply eating less. The logical thing is to cut down on high-fat, high-sugar and high-calorie foods, especially if they are low in protein, vitamins and minerals. Think of it this way. One pound of fat provides about 3,500 calories; to lose that you will therefore need to consume 3,500 calories fewer than usual. You can do that in a week by simply reducing your daily intake by 500 calories.

For average Nods a crash diet is a real no-no. Although your calorie intake may be minimal and the pounds come off quickly, it is not just the blubber that's melting away. You also lose a lot of water and muscle. Once you start to eat normally again the weight piles on faster than you shed it. Yo-yo dieting – repeated weight loss and regain – is, in the long run, actually much more dangerous to your health than being a stable porker.

The most effective way to lose fat and retain muscle is do so gradually, no more than 1-2 lb a week. Aerobic exercise – like cycling and jogging – burns off fat and whacks up your metabolic rate for a short time after a 'sesh' (Marine slang for an exercise session).

What is important is the type of food we eat. As your training schedule increases in intensity you will be burning up more and more calories. Fat will be burned off and replaced by muscle – which is heavier – but you can help this process along. It's no good doing a 45-minute running circuit if as soon as you feel hungry you consume a Mars Bar coated in batter, deep fried and served with chips. Please, if you have to have batter at least make sure it has fresh fish or a banana inside!

Unfortunately many people's diets are destined to kill them because they contain so much cholesterol which can harm, fur up or generally block the arteries. It makes sense to avoid cholesterol-rich foods. It is also vital to be at the very least aware of what you are eating. You do not put diesel fuel into a petrol driven car. Of course, not everyone has the same metabolism. Some people convert food into fuel incredibly fast, and never seem to put on weight no matter what they eat.

Generally, we all eat too much because we can. Think about the last really good meal you ate. Remember the point at which you thought 'I'm full, that was great and I don't need these last two mouthfuls'. But you ate them anyway. Try eating because you are hungry and stop when you have had enough.

Another trick is to try to change not only what and how much you eat but also when and how often. When in serious training, many athletes will divide their food intake into five or six meals a day, never leaving an interval of more than three hours between each meal. For most working people this is imprac- tical but we can learn from it, perhaps by changing the balance of the meals. In order to speed up putting on extra pounds Japanese Sumo wrestlers like to have a huge meal followed by a sleep. Reversing that theory, it is better not to have your main meal at night as you have less time to burn any of it off. Eat a lighter supper and a bigger breakfast: you consume the same amount of calories but give your body more chance to burn them off.

As you undergo the Nod Circuit Programme, you may well find you need to eat more, especially mid-morning or at teatime. That's no problem – have a snack. But make sure it's a muesli not a Mars Bar, carrot sticks or a banana, not a cream bun. If you have an established eating routine, do not skip meals or go for long periods of time without eating. This might lead to low blood sugar levels which will make your feet feel like lead during exercise.

Your Calorie Intake

As with any highly refined and tuned machine the excessive input of a partic- ular type of foodstuff can do harm, so don't over-indulge in one type of food but rather try to maintain a balance. Most seasonal foodstuffs, especially fruit, vegetables and salads are now available all year round.

You should aim to get 45-65 per cent of your total calorie intake from car- bohydrates, preferably in the form of complex carbohydrates (starchy foods like bread, pasta and potatoes). Eating a carbohydrate-dominated diet should not be expensive, whereas buying ready-made meals, or other so-called 'convenience foods' is a waste of money. A ready-made lasagne costs twice as much as a home-made one and very rarely tastes as good. Also, many ready-made foods are often very high in calories compared to fresh ingredients.

What it always comes down to is time – not taste. It's so much easier to shove a frozen lasagne in the microwave. Yes, food is fuel but it can also be a source of great pleasure. If you are prepared to try a different diet you must also be prepared to take a little bit of extra effort to make it taste nice. It isn't difficult… and the results are generally very worth while.

What about drink?

Drink as much as you need and want – provided it's **not** alcohol. Water is the best of all liquids to consume. Current medical research has it that a little alcohol is good for you but too much is very bad. It has been shown that red wine in moderate quantities (one to two glasses a day) can aid the immune system and help to reduce heart disease. Unfortunately alcohol does not improve any aspect of physical performance. Endurance, speed, strength and stamina may actually suffer. Most serious athletes avoid large quantities of booze.

Alcohol before a training session is not recommended because of the effect it has on the body. It slows the thought processes – making you unco-ordinated – and increases blood pressure and cardiac output. Another of booze's adverse effects is that it's a diuretic; you end up peeing too much and get dehydrated. Before a session make sure you have had plenty of fluids. (Check the colour of your urine – the yellower it is the more dehydrated you are.) Always have a bottle of water to hand during exercise, and stop regularly for a sip of water. When you have finished, top up any fluid loss.

There is now an enormous variety of sports drinks on the market. These claim to help the athlete by either boosting the carbohydrate content or replacing the electrolytes (salts and minerals) lost during a workout. Some scientific tests do show an improvement in certain conditions but the jury is still out. Despite their name, electrolytes do not shock the body into improving its performance; what they do is speed up water delivery to the body.

There are three types of sports drinks – hypotonic, isotonic and hyper-tonic. Hypotonic fluids (eg Dexter's, Replay, NesFit) are less concentrated than body fluids and so are absorbed into the body faster than water. Isotonic drinks (Lucozade Sports, Gatorade, Isostar) have the same concentration of

Make your own sports drinks

You can make your own sports drinks at a fraction of the cost of the commercial variety.

Hypotonic	Isotonic	Hypertonic
20 g glucose or sucrose	50 g glucose/sucrose	100 g glucose/sucrose
1 litre warm water	1 litre warm water	1 litre warm water
good pinch salt	good pinch salt	good pinch salt

Dissolve the sugar and salt in the water, allow to cool and keep cold in the fridge.

or

Hypotonic	Isotonic	Hypertonic
250 ml unsweetened juice	500 ml unsweetened juice	1 litre unsweetened juice
750 ml water	500 ml water	
good pinch salt	good pinch salt	good pinch salt

Mix all the ingredients together and keep cold.

or

Hypotonic	Isotonic	Hypertonic
100 ml fruit squash	200 ml fruit squash	400 ml fruit squash
1 litre water	1 litre water	1 litre water
good pinch salt	good pinch salt	good pinch salt

Mix all the ingredients together and keep cold.

Any fruit juice – pineapple, apple, orange, grapefruit or a mixture – will do provided it is unsweetened. The fruit creates fructose which is a natural sugar. Salt can be increased or decreased depending on your taste but do not omit it altogether.

dissolved particles as body fluids and will therefore be absorbed at the same, or slightly faster, pace as water. Hypertonic fluids are more concentrated and are thus absorbed slowly. Drinks like Ultra Fuel and Top Form contain extra carbohydrate and claim they can give an energy boost. Hypertonics tend to be better if you have exercised for more than two hours.

Smoking and exercise

Medical reports on the problems associated with smoking are well known and documented. Aside from the fact that smoking a packet of cigarettes a day doubles the risk of heart disease, when a smoker takes part in any kind of physical exercise his performance is impaired because his body requires more oxygen and his heart beats faster.

If you are a smoker and don't want to give up that is your choice. However, certainly in the initial stages of training, you will find some of the exercises much harder if you smoke. This might be the perfect reason you need to give up fags for good.

SCRAN (NUTRITION)

The Next Step

Right, that's the lecture over. No doubt you've heard it a million times and don't need it. Fair enough. It's your choice. But don't forget that you control your body, what you eat and what exercise you take. This is a suggested diet plan for the first two weeks, with possible menus for seven days (repeat with variations during the second week). Nothing in it requires the abilities of a Michelin chef to prepare … but remember real food tastes better than pre-packaged – whatever the adverts say. The quantities you consume will depend on your workload. Cutting down food consumption will result in weight loss but be careful. Reduce the quantities at each meal gradually and try to increase your exercise rate and frequency. There are certain people who if they are exercising more might actually need to put on weight. If you are one of these people then you must consider increasing your food intake (but sticking with the good stuff) as your exercise rate goes up.

Just one last thing. For the first two weeks all alcohol and cigarettes are banned. You have made one commitment to get fit. Now make another.

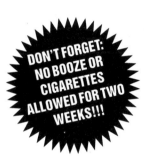

DON'T FORGET: NO BOOZE OR CIGARETTES ALLOWED FOR TWO WEEKS!!!

DAY 1

Breakfast 2 Weetabix with semi-skimmed milk, teaspoon of sugar/ sweetener ● 2 slices wholemeal toast, with butter substitute, marmalade ● Apple or banana

Lunch Baked potato with canned tuna and cheese filling ● Salad (without the mayonnaise) ● Fresh fruit

Dinner Spaghetti Bolognese (use lean mince) ● Ice cream (low fat) and fruit

DAY 2

Breakfast Poached egg on wholemeal toast ● 2 slices wholemeal toast, with butter substitute ● Fresh fruit

Lunch Soup (canned or fresh) ● Bread/ roll ● Fresh fruit

Dinner Casserole with baked potatoes ● Cheese (low fat) and biscuits

DAY 3

Breakfast Grilled bacon, baked beans ● 2 slices wholemeal toast, with butter substitute ● Tomatoes and 2 poached eggs

Lunch Fish (tuna/sardines. Not in batter!) and salad ● Oven chips or baked potato ● Fresh fruit

Dinner   Roast chicken (without skin) ● Baked potatoes or steamed rice ● Greens and carrots ● Fresh fruit

DAY 4

Breakfast   Yogurt (low fat) with fresh fruit chopped in ● 2 slices wholemeal toast, with butter substitute

Lunch   Baked beans on 2 slices wholemeal toast

Dinner   Lasagne (low-fat cheese) with French bread ● Salad ● Low-fat rice pudding

DAY 5

Breakfast   Kippers and poached egg ● 2 slices wholemeal toast, with butter substitute ● Apple or banana

Lunch   Baked potato with chicken and sweetcorn filling ● Coleslaw and tomatoes ● Fresh fruit

Dinner   Shepherd's pie (lean mince) ● Steamed or *al dente* vegetables ● Fresh fruit

DAY 6

Breakfast   2 Weetabix with semi-skimmed milk, teaspoon of sugar/ sweetener ● 2 slices wholemeal toast, with butter substitute, marmalade ● Apple or banana

Lunch   Minestrone soup ● Salad ● Fresh fruit

Dinner   Grilled fish (mackerel or salmon steak) ● Lentils with onion and carrot ● Ice cream (low fat)

DAY 7

Breakfast   Pink grapefruit (no sugar) ● 3 slices wholemeal toast, with butter substitute, marmalade

Lunch   Cottage cheese (low fat), raw vegetable salad ● Wholemeal roll ● Fresh fruit

Dinner   Paella (chicken, fish, vegetables) ● Fruit

All Week

Beverages

Tea/coffee with semi-skimmed milk (try to reduce sugar intake)

Water has no calories – try to drink 2 litres a day

Fruit juices – even unsweetened juices – have natural sugars so dilute with water

Snacks

Fresh fruit (especially apples and bananas)

Raw vegetables (carrots etc)

Power bars and muesli bars

Important Note

After the first two weeks, plan your diet so you eat as much good scran and as little bad scran as possible.

Bad Scran: Cholesterol Nasties

Try to avoid these foods:

Fatty red meats ● Egg yolks ● Dairy products made from full-fat milk (butter, yogurt, cheese) ● Fried foods – especially those fried in animal fat ● Poultry skin ● Foods with lots of refined sugar – cakes, sweets, biscuits etc.

Good Scran: Carb Power

Carbohydrates tend to be much cheaper than proteins and are better for you as they don't have high levels of cholesterol and harmful fats.

Pasta ● Pulses ● Rice ● Potatoes ● Brown bread ● Fresh fruit ● Beans/ peas ● Cereals

Warming Up, Cooling Down and Stretching

Everyone today is in a constant hurry. Instant communication has given us less time for leisure activities, not more. So we want to get on with whatever we are doing as quickly as possible because we all have less time to do the things we want – or rather what we think we want – to do.

'Look I'm pushed for time, I'm already fit, let's just get on with it shall we? I'm not going to stretch my legs like some poncey ballet dancer. Warming up is for wimps.' We've heard that, or variations of it, a million times and the men who say it are fools. One day the idiots are going to scream because they are going to be in pain. And it serves them right.

Let's look at Joe, our less than average circuit trainer. First he drives the mile to the gym, that saves vital time, you see. While getting changed he warms up by chatting about the 'sesh' – which only warms his throat. He dives straight into the first exercise with a rush of adrenaline. His heartbeat instantly races to within coronary range. His muscles scream in pain. By the seventh dip he's suffering from acute breathlessness which impairs any ability to perform properly. His flexibility is nil – he's as supple as a chocolate frog but nowhere near as attractive to passing princesses. By the time he's four sit-ups into the second exercise he's not so much hanging out as swinging from a gibbet. And it's going to get worse.

The reason for all this unnecessary pain is that Joe has not done a proper, constructive, structured warm-up. Tackling hard exercise without a proper warm-up is akin to getting married after the first date – fraught with risks and doomed to failure.

Look at this way. If your car has been sitting under three feet of snow for a week, you don't just hack a tunnel to the driver's door, leap in, turn on the ignition and expect the machine to accelerate from 0-60 in 10 seconds. You expect it to blow up – if it starts at all. Warming up just means getting your engine running smoothly, making sure that all the working parts are lubricated, that there is water in the radiator and enough petrol in the tank. An Olympic sprinter will warm up for anything between 45-60 minutes for a race that may only last 10 seconds. Doesn't that tell you something?

Exercise without a proper warm-up will lead – at best – to poor performance and – at worst – to injury.

A warm-up is designed to increase steadily the blood flow to the muscles and raise the body temperature. This, in turn, warms the muscles and assists them in contracting easily, enhancing the ability to produce strength and speed. It's also a great way of warming up a body that is about to be beasted. A warmed-up muscle is a more efficient muscle in every way.

Warming up also promotes the flow of synovial fluid to the joints – naturally lubricating a rusty hinge – which improves flexibility during exercise. This is very important for circuit training. In order to perform the exercises correctly, and thereby improve your strength and flexibility, you must go through the proper range of movement in all the exercises.

Marine recruits start their physical training with a 15-week course of thrice weekly Swedish PT exercises. A good five-minute warm-up is always done before a severe hour-long workout. It's just in later life they forget and PTIs have seen many a Marine limp away from an individual 'sesh' halfway through, because of a muscle strain. The bottom line is that warming up will make the transition from a simple effort to hard exercise very much easier and will also reduce the risk of injury.

For professional athletes, stretching is a natural process they go through almost without thinking – both before and after exercise. To part-timers it's often the boring bit before the action – and afterwards they're too shattered to bother. But they change their attitude once they have worked out the direct relationship between not stretching (or mobilising) and the subsequent **pain**.

One of the components which makes up physical fitness is FLEXIBILITY – the ability to flex and extend the joint through its normal range of movement. This is specific to each joint and most people's joints have the potential to move through a larger range of motion than the surrounding muscles will allow. By stretching regularly, the muscle's capacities are extended, thereby giving the joint a greater range of motion. Being flexible improves general body mobility and awareness, making routine tasks easier and helping to improve your posture. It helps to reduce the risk of injury, the incidence of lower back pain and muscle soreness. It also assists in improving performance and technique. The major cause of declining flexibility is lack of movement.

The message is simple. Use it or lose it.

Warming up for your circuit

Your warm-up should be seen as an integral part of the workout, not as an annoying prelude. It has four parts: warm-up exercises, mobilising exercises, stretches and a re-warm. Most of the circuits in this book have been designed to be completed in just over half an hour. If you have only 30 minutes to train, don't miss the warm-up but structure your workout like this:

> 5 minutes warm-up (eg 3 minutes skipping/jogging plus
> 2 minutes stretching)
> 20 minutes sesh
> 5 minutes cool-down (eg 2 minutes slow jogging plus
> 3 minutes stretching)

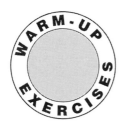

Warm-up exercises

These are designed to warm up different parts of the body and increase the heart rate and overall body temperature. Incorporate as many exercises as time allows. Remember that you should be warming up your whole body (don't forget the Whole Body Approach).

BALANCING

Walk along a bench, follow a line etc, gathering speed if possible (this will help to sharpen reactions). Hold your arms out like a tightrope-walker to help keep your balance.

JOGGING ON THE SPOT

Keep the body upright and knees soft – or take the lock off the knees as they say in the Marines.

DORSAL RAISES

Lie face down, with hands clasped behind back. Raise head, shoulders, chest and legs off floor. Lower, and repeat.

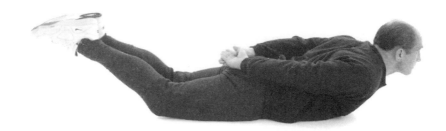

BUM KICKS

Jog on the spot and kick heels up behind, aiming to touch backside.

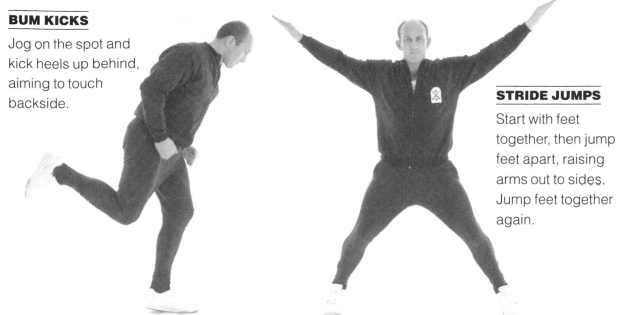

STRIDE JUMPS

Start with feet together, then jump feet apart, raising arms out to sides. Jump feet together again.

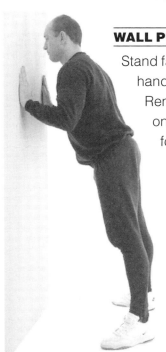

WALL PUSHES

Stand facing wall. Place both hands on wall and push away. Remember to put hands back on the wall on the way forwards.

STEP-UPS

Use a step or box. Step up with right foot, then bring left foot up to join it. Step back down with right foot, then follow with left foot. Make sure you place the whole of the foot on the box as you step up.

SKIPPING

Without a rope – like a kid going to school.

SPLIT JUMPS

Jump and land with one leg forwards, one leg back. Jump again and switch position of legs.

WARMING UP, COOLING DOWN AND STRETCHING

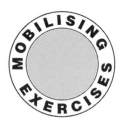

Mobilising exercises

These incorporate gentle rhythmic movements which take the joints through their full range of movement. In addition to the exercises illustrated here, do the following as well:

NECK MOBILISATION

Turn the neck side to side, up and down (not backwards).

SHOULDER SHRUGGING

Raise both shoulders towards ears, then lower them again. This helps to loosen the shoulder area.

SWIMMING STROKES

Do front crawl, back crawl and breaststroke arm movements through the air.

WRIST FLEXING

Hold on to one arm and move wrist up and down. Repeat with other wrist.

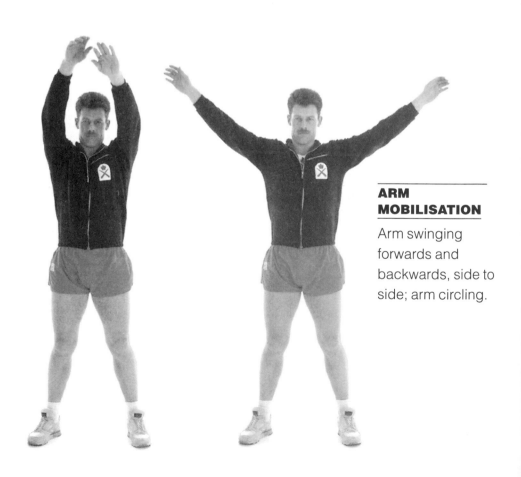

ARM MOBILISATION

Arm swinging forwards and backwards, side to side; arm circling.

HIP MOBILISATION

Hip swaying side to side; forwards and backwards; hip circling.

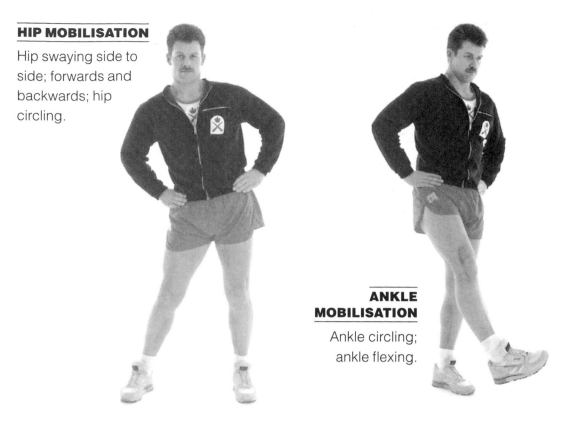

ANKLE MOBILISATION

Ankle circling; ankle flexing.

TOE TOUCHING

With feet hip-width or shoulder-width apart (depending on your flexibility), touch alternate hands to toes.

KNEE BENDING

Keep knees over feet as you alternately bend and straighten knees.

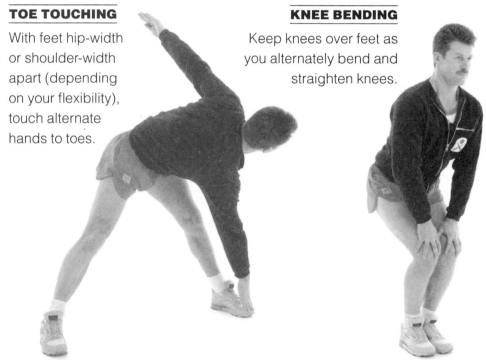

Towards the end of the mobilising sesh start to speed up the exercises.

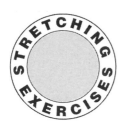

Stretching

Before you move on to the circuit training exercises, it is important to stretch out the main muscle groups you will be using. Warming up the muscles in this way will make them more pliable and less susceptible to injury. Likewise, at the end of your workout, stretching out the main muscle groups you have been using will help to dissipate waste products and lactic acid that build up in the muscles during exercise, and also reduce the likelihood of soreness.

After your workout, while the muscles are still warm, is also a good time to work on increasing your flexibility. Specific strengthening exercises can sometimes cause the muscles to shorten and, in turn, restrict their range of movement, which results in a decrease in flexibility. Therefore, in order to maintain or increase flexibility in the joints as well as reduce the risk of injury, it's important to include an effective stretching routine, one which uses a combined stretching and relaxation technique, at the end of each workout.

Keep it simple

Use the static stretching method – the stretch and hold technique – where the position is assumed slowly and gently and then held for the required length of time. We use three stretching routines: Easy, Intermediate and Advanced. Start with the easy stretches and progress to the more difficult ones. Gradually, try to increase the length of time you hold each stretch.

Ten golden rules for stretching

1 Ensure you are in the correct starting position.
2 Breathe naturally – never hold your breath.
3 Always release the stretch SLOWLY.
4 Joints should be in alignment in all standing stretches – shoulders above hips, hips above knees, knees above ankles.
5 **Never** bounce. This causes an unnatural elasticity in the muscles and can lead to injury.
6 **Never** ask a friend to push the stretch further (this is a specialised form of stretching).
7 Hold the stretch for a minimum of 10 seconds when warming up and 20 seconds when cooling down or working on improving flexibility.
8 Relax under control.
9 Stretch each muscle group once only per each stretching session.
10 Take a whole body approach (WBA) and stretch all major muscle groups.

It's advisable to stretch at least **once** a day, even on the days you are not exercising. And for the stretches to be of proper benefit, you must perform them **correctly**. So, make a habit of stretching for 10 minutes every day. Always work from the head downwards, or the feet upwards.

Before exercising, hold each stretch for 10 seconds.

After exercising, hold each stretch for 20-30 seconds. When the sensation eases in the muscle, try to increase the stretch a little to develop your flexibility further.

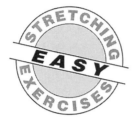

WEEKS 1-2

TRICEP STRETCH

- Stand with feet hip-width apart, knees soft. Place palm of one hand flat between your shoulder blades, elbow pointing upwards. Bring other arm over your head, placing hand on top of elbow. Keeping shoulders pulled back, gently push down with top hand, and hold.
- Swap arms and repeat.

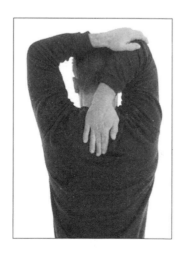

When not to stretch

It is advisable not to stretch if ...
- A bone blocks motion.
- You've had a recent fracture.
- You sustain a sharp pain during joint movement or muscle stretch.
- You've had a recent sprain or injury.
- There is a loss of function or a decrease in the range of movement.

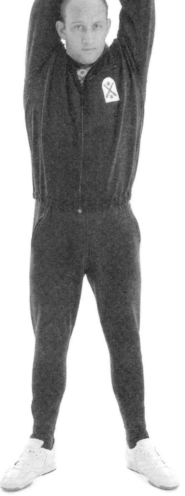

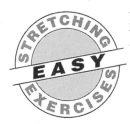

SHOULDER STRETCH

- Place one arm across your chest and bring other arm up, bent, to press on right tricep (back of upper arm) of arm across chest. Hold.
- Swap arms and repeat.

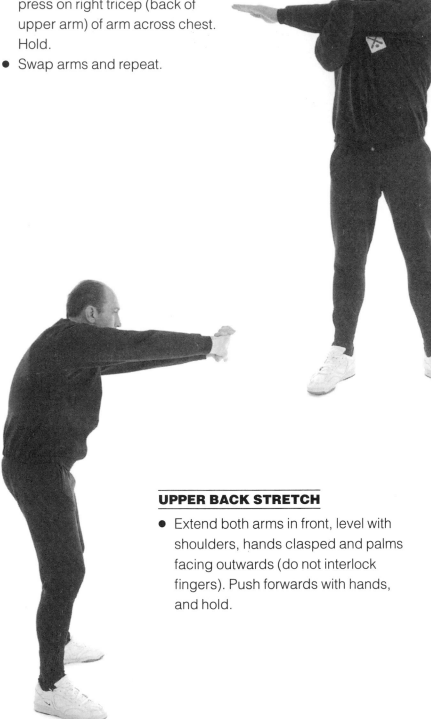

UPPER BACK STRETCH

- Extend both arms in front, level with shoulders, hands clasped and palms facing outwards (do not interlock fingers). Push forwards with hands, and hold.

WARMING UP, COOLING DOWN AND STRETCHING

CHEST STRETCH

- Clasp hands behind back (do not interlock fingers). Raise arms as high as you can, and hold. Keep body as upright as possible.

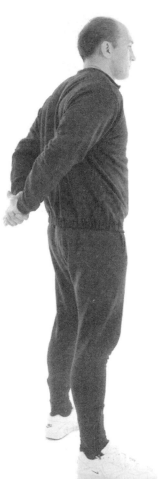

SIDE STRETCH

- Sit on the floor with soles of feet together or legs comfortably crossed. Place one hand on floor and reach up and over with other arm. Hold.
- Repeat to other side.

LYING QUAD STRETCH

- Lie on your side and prop yourself up on your elbow. Take hold of the ankle of the top leg and pull it towards your backside to stretch front of thigh. Hold.
- Roll over, and repeat with other leg.

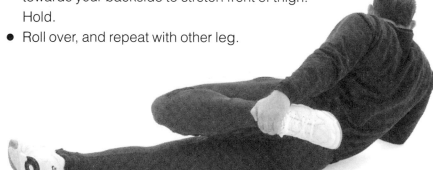

WARMING UP, COOLING DOWN AND STRETCHING

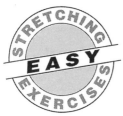

LYING HAMSTRING STRETCH

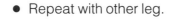

- Lie on your back, with one leg relaxed. Bend other knee in towards chest and take hold of calf with both hands. Slowly pull leg towards you, trying to straighten it as much as possible. Hold. Release the leg, bend it and slowly lower it to floor.
- Repeat with other leg.

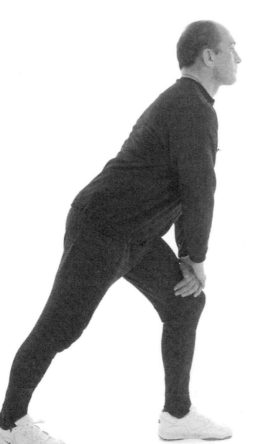

CALF STRETCH

- Stand with one leg in front of the other and both feet pointing forwards. Place hands on front thigh. Keeping your back straight and both feet flat on the floor, slowly bend front knee until you feel a sensation in the calf muscle of back leg. Hold. To increase the stretch, lean further over front leg.
- Swap legs and repeat.

WEEKS 3–6

In addition to the exercises illustrated here, also do the following as in Weeks 1-3:

TRICEP STRETCH

(see page 31)

UPPER BACK STRETCH

(see page 32)

SIDE STRETCH

- Stand with feet wide apart, knees soft, and feet pointing forwards. Place one hand on thigh and, without leaning forwards or backwards or locking the knees, reach up and over with other arm, and hold.
- Repeat to other side.

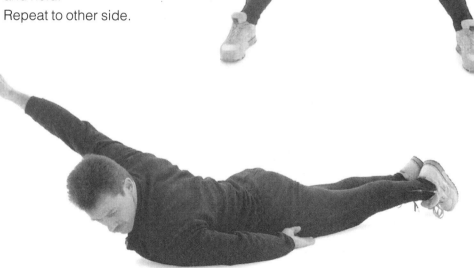

LYING SHOULDER STRETCH

- Lie face down on the floor and place one arm by your side. Stretch other arm out in front, with fingers stretched. Lift the outstretched arm off floor, and hold. Slowly release the stretch and return arm to floor.
- Swap arms and repeat.

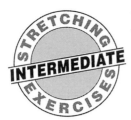
LYING CHEST STRETCH

- Still lying face down, clasp hands behind your back (do not interlock fingers). Lift arms until you feel a sensation in your chest, and hold.

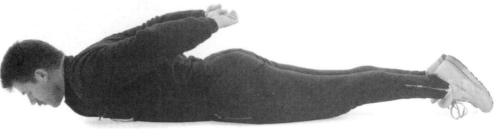

ELONGATION

- Lie on your back and extend arms and legs. Point toes and stretch fingers, and hold.

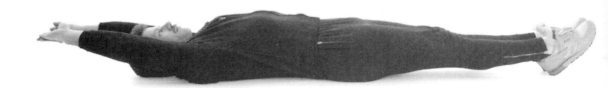

SEAT STRETCH

- Still lying on your back, with head on floor, legs extended and your lower back flat, use hands to pull one knee towards chest until you feel a sensation in your back and the back of the raised leg. Hold. Slowly release leg.
- Repeat with other leg.

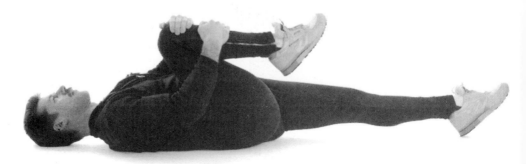

GROIN STRETCH

- Sit upright with soles of feet together. Use your elbows to gently press knees towards floor. Hold.

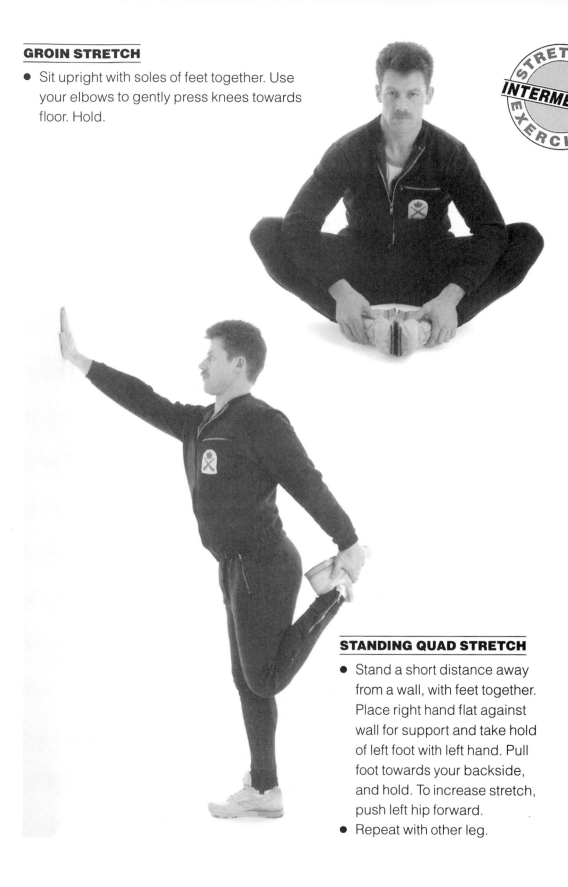

STANDING QUAD STRETCH

- Stand a short distance away from a wall, with feet together. Place right hand flat against wall for support and take hold of left foot with left hand. Pull foot towards your backside, and hold. To increase stretch, push left hip forward.
- Repeat with other leg.

WARMING UP, COOLING DOWN AND STRETCHING

37

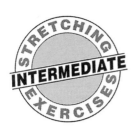

STANDING HAMSTRING STRETCH

- Standing away from the wall, bend right knee and push left foot straight out in front of you until you feel a mild sensation in the back of the left thigh. Hold.
- Swap legs and repeat.

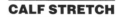

CALF STRETCH

- Stand a short distance away from wall, with one leg in front of other leg, so that both feet are pointing forwards. Place both hands on wall for support and, keeping your back straight and both feet flat on the floor, bend front knee until you feel a sensation in the calf muscle of back leg. Hold. To increase the stretch, lean further over front leg.
  - Swap legs and repeat.

WARMING UP, COOLING DOWN AND STRETCHING

WEEKS 7–8

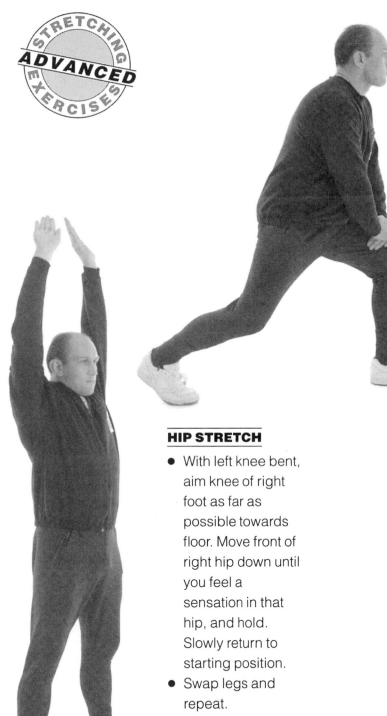

STRETCHING ADVANCED EXERCISES

In addition to the exercises illustrated here, also do the following as in Weeks 1-6:

TRICEP STRETCH

(see page 31)

UPPER BACK STRETCH

(see page 32)

CHEST STRETCH

(see page 33)

SIDE STRETCH

(see page 35)

GROIN STRETCH

(see page 37)

CALF STRETCH

(see page 34)

SHOULDER STRETCH

- Extend both arms straight above head. Breathe in as you stretch arms up and back, and hold.

HIP STRETCH

- With left knee bent, aim knee of right foot as far as possible towards floor. Move front of right hip down until you feel a sensation in that hip, and hold. Slowly return to starting position.
- Swap legs and repeat.

WARMING UP, COOLING DOWN AND STRETCHING

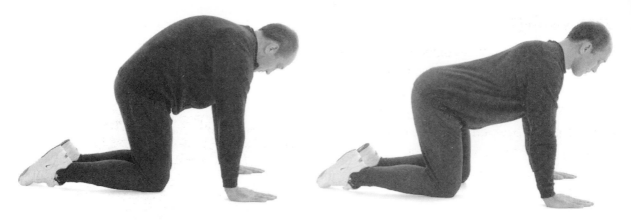

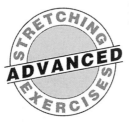

CAT STRETCH

- To stretch the shoulders, arms and broad back muscles, position yourself on hands and knees on the floor. Arch the back upwards until you feel a sensation in the back, and hold. Now press the back flat until you feel a sensation, and hold.

CHEST AND SHOULDER STRETCH

- Stand by a wall (or fence) with feet wide apart. Place one hand against the wall at shoulder level, with arm outstretched. Turn away from outstretched arm but keep shoulder pressed against the wall. You will feel a sensation in the chest and shoulder region. Hold, then relax.
- Repeat with other arm.

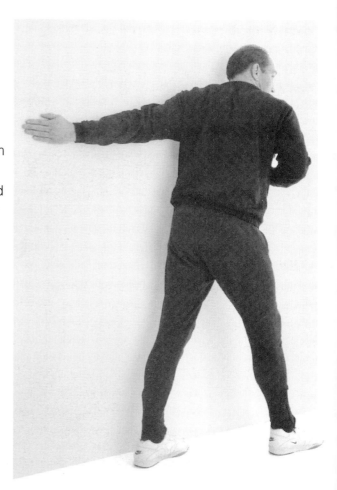

SPINE TWISTER

- Sit upright with right leg extended. Bend left leg and cross it over right leg. Rest left arm against inside of left thigh, just above the knee. Using left elbow to keep left leg still, slowly twist upper body to left while turning head to look over left shoulder. Hold. Slowly return to starting position.
- Swap legs and repeat to other side.

SITTING HAMSTRING STRETCH

- Sitting upright, extend right leg and place left sole against right thigh. Reach towards ankle (do not grasp ankle) by bending forwards from hips until you feel a sensation in the back of right thigh. Hold. Slowly return to starting position.
- Swap legs and repeat.

STRETCHING **ADVANCED** EXERCISES

LYING QUAD STRETCH

- Lie on your side and prop yourself up on your elbow. Take hold of the ankle of the top leg and pull it towards your backside to stretch front of thigh. Hold.
- Roll over, and repeat with other leg.

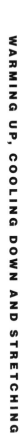

WARMING UP, COOLING DOWN AND STRETCHING

Run Throughs/Re-warms

When you have finished these basic mobilisation and stretching exercises, go through heart-rate-raising exercises again but faster. Go all the way through your intended circuit once. Repeat each exercise three times SLOWLY. This has two advantages. It is a rehearsal to get the exercise right. It's also a specific warm-up related to the workout so you know you are warming the correct muscles. Finish with 10 good tuck jumps (see page 76) or a short sprint to get really psyched up. (If you are doing a sports specific circuit use the ball during this period or mimic the actions of the sport at an increased tempo.)

In circuit training the warm-up should immediately precede the workout, so prepare the circuit before you warm up. Then don't hang about letting your body cool down. Get straight in there.

ALWAYS WARM UP

Important tips

- It is essential that you warm up in the same environment that you are planning to exercise in. If it's a cold crisp winter day and you're planning a 30-minute run, don't cop out and do the warm-up inside your nice cosy home. If you do, the chances are that the shock of the cold will seize up some of your muscles. The bad news is that in cold weather – because you are trying to raise your body temperature – the warm-up will have to be longer to reach the required level. Before cross-country ski races in Norway, Marines spend at least one hour stretching, mobilising and then skiing in order to prepare for the race.
- The more intense the workout you plan, the more intense the warm-up should be. If you are about to sprint 100 metres, the warm-up should include some fast sprints before the race. If you are about to undertake a marathon, a long slow, steady, progressive warm-up is needed.
- The earlier in the day you start exercising, the longer the warm-up you need to do. Don't leap straight out of bed, touch your toes twice and run a mile.
- And now for some good news. The fitter you are, the less time you require to warm up. But remember that even the professionals warm up.

Cooling Down

All physical activity should finish with a cool-down – the opposite of a warm-up. Imagine you have been running a series of 400-metre sprints. Your heart is pumped up, your muscles are primed. Then you just stop. Although you feel relief initially, remember that your muscles which have been working at full capacity have been ordered to stand still. It's like driving a car at 100 mph on the motorway, then slamming on the brakes and driving it in high gear at 10 mph. The engine doesn't like it. It may not be today or tomorrow but it will complain one day – when it is most inconvenient.

By lowering the intensity of the exercise the circulatory system is gradually brought back to your pre-exercise state, which prevents the risk of fainting or dizziness. It helps dissipate the build-up of waste products such as lactic acid which can cause stiffness and soreness.

If you follow these cool-down exercises with a series of relaxing exercises (such as breathing deeply or a few mobilising exercises carried out really slowly), tension and stress will be reduced and flexibility increased. In other words you will not just be ready but raring to face the rest of the day.

The Cool-down

Once you have finished exercising, your body temperature must be reduced gradually, and your heart rate allowed to slow down naturally. Easy jogging and walking will suffice and as the intensity decreases then you should perform a series of easy mobilising exercises such as swinging your arms, and knee bends. You can repeat the warm-up exercises at a reduced intensity.

You should follow this with a short series of longer developmental stretches. Cool-down stretches are the same as warm-up stretches but they are held for longer – 20-30 seconds as opposed to 10 in the warm-up before the circuit. Choose the main muscle groups immediately after the cool-down and do a few stretches on minor muscle groups. The main muscle groups are the hamstrings (back thighs), quadriceps (front thighs), pectorals (chest), latissimus dorsi (upper back) and gastrocnemius (calf muscles). The minor ones are the shoulder muscles (deltoids), forearms (flexors and extensors), side (obliques), and arms (triceps and biceps). A developmental stretch should also last 20-30 seconds. When you feel a sensation in the muscle group, try to stretch a little further, then hold and relax. This increases flexibility.

Finally do a few relaxing exercises (breathing deeply and some mobilising exercises done slowly) followed by a quick wake-up burst (knee lifts or running on the spot) so you finish on a high.

WARMING UP, COOLING DOWN AND STRETCHING

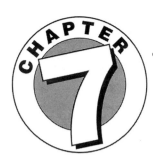

The Circuit Exercises

Here are the main circuit exercises that are used throughout this book. It's a good idea to familiarise yourself with these before launching yourself into the Circuit Programme. An index is provided on page 144 so that you can quickly refer back if necessary.

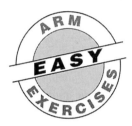

Arm Exercises: Easy

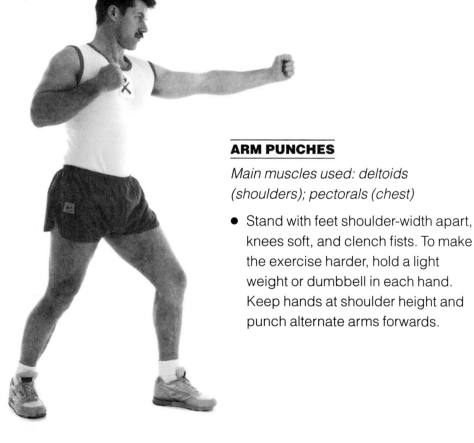

ARM PUNCHES

Main muscles used: deltoids (shoulders); pectorals (chest)

- Stand with feet shoulder-width apart, knees soft, and clench fists. To make the exercise harder, hold a light weight or dumbbell in each hand. Keep hands at shoulder height and punch alternate arms forwards.

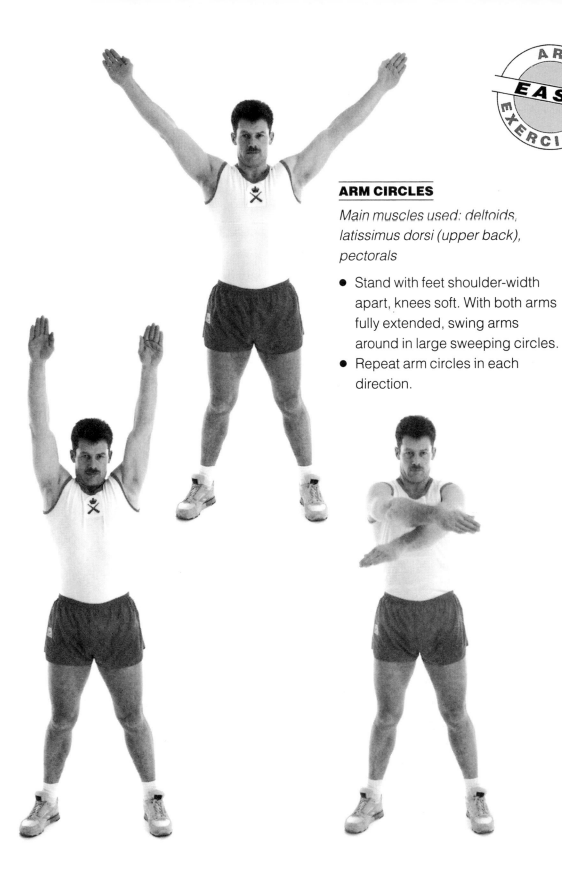

ARM CIRCLES

Main muscles used: deltoids, latissimus dorsi (upper back), pectorals

- Stand with feet shoulder-width apart, knees soft. With both arms fully extended, swing arms around in large sweeping circles.
- Repeat arm circles in each direction.

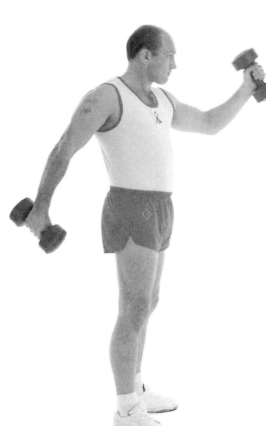

ARM SWINGS

Main muscles used: deltoids; pectorals

- Stand with feet shoulder-width apart, knees soft. Hold a light weight or dumbbell in each hand. Bend arms and swing alternate arms forwards and backwards with *control*.

SHOULDER SHRUGS

Main muscles used: trapezius (back of shoulders); deltoids

- Stand with feet hip-width apart, knees soft, and hold a light weight or dumbbell in each hand.
- Keep arms close by your sides and shrug shoulders, bringing them up towards your ears. Release and repeat.

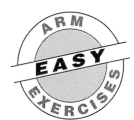

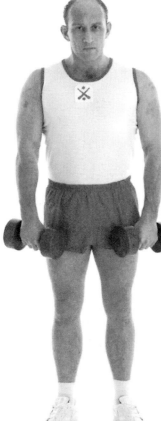

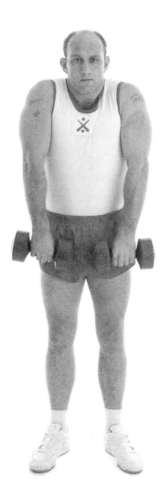

WRIST CURLS

Main muscles used: flexors and extensors of forearms

- Sit on a bench or chair, with your feet wide apart, and grip a dumbbell tightly in right hand. Rest right elbow on knee.
- Keeping right elbow as still as possible, flex right wrist upwards. Return to starting position and repeat.
- Swap arms and repeat. Do an equal number of reps with each wrist.

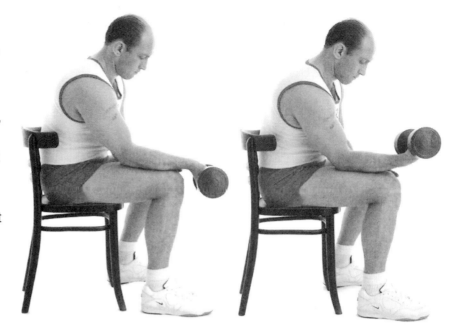

WEIGHT WINDING ON ROPE

Main muscles used: forearms; deltoids (statically)

For this exercise you will need a small bar or pole that can be held in both hands. Tie it to a piece of rope, and have a small weight (or a kilo bag of sugar inside a separate plastic bag will do) suspended from the bar.

- Standing with feet shoulder-width apart, knees soft, hold the bar with both hands, using either an underhand or overhand grip. Wind the rope so that the weight comes up towards the bar, then unwind the rope to lower the weight gently.
- Repeat.

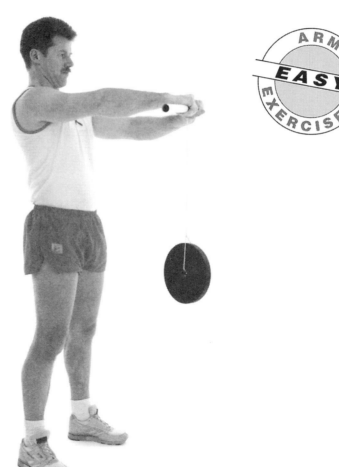

ARM EASY EXERCISES

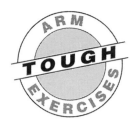

Arm Exercises: Tough

DIPS

Main muscles used: deltoids; triceps (back of upper arm)

This exercise is best performed on a bench because it is much more stable, but you can also do it using a chair if you haven't a bench to hand.

- Sit on the edge of the chair, with hands facing forwards and resting on the edge of the seat. Keeping knees bent and feet flat on floor, move your upper body and knees forwards so that your backside comes off chair and your weight is supported on your hands.

- Using the strength of your arms to support you, flex your elbows so that your backside is lowered towards, but does not touch, floor.
- Straighten your arms (but do not lock elbows) to raise yourself up again, and repeat.

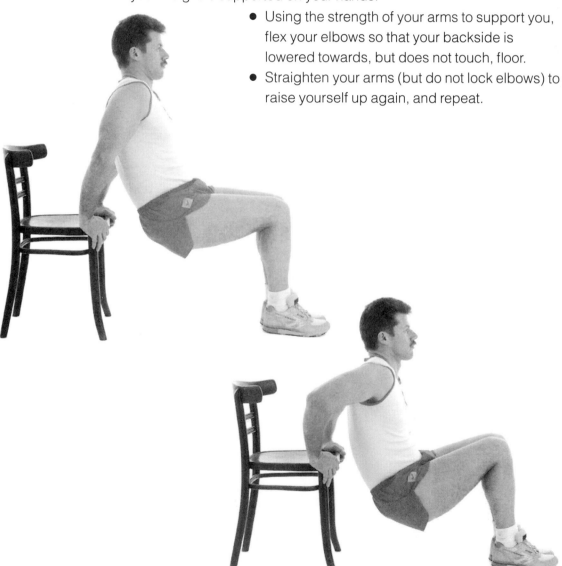

TRICEP PRESSES

Main muscles used: triceps

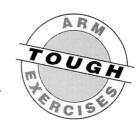

- Stand with your back straight and feet hip-width apart, knees soft. Hold a light weight or dumbbell in your right hand. Bring right elbow close to your head and place the weight or dumbbell between your shoulder blades, and place your left hand on your chest.
- Keeping right elbow as still as possible, extend right forearm up towards ceiling, raising the weight or dumbbell as high as you can. Take care not to lock the elbow.
- Bring forearm back down so that the weight or dumbbell rests once more between your shoulder blades. Repeat.
- Repeat with left arm, making sure you do an equal number of reps with each arm.

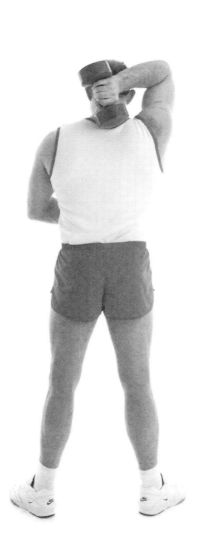

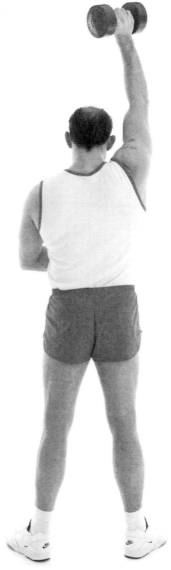

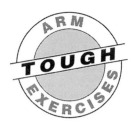

ALTERNATE SHOULDER PRESSES

Main muscles used: deltoids; triceps; upper pectorals

- Stand with feet shoulder-width apart, knees soft, and hold a light weight or dumbbell in each hand. Bend arms and place weights at top of chest.
- Without locking elbow, straighten one arm upwards, then lower weight to top of chest.
- Repeat with other arm, and continue to raise alternate arms.

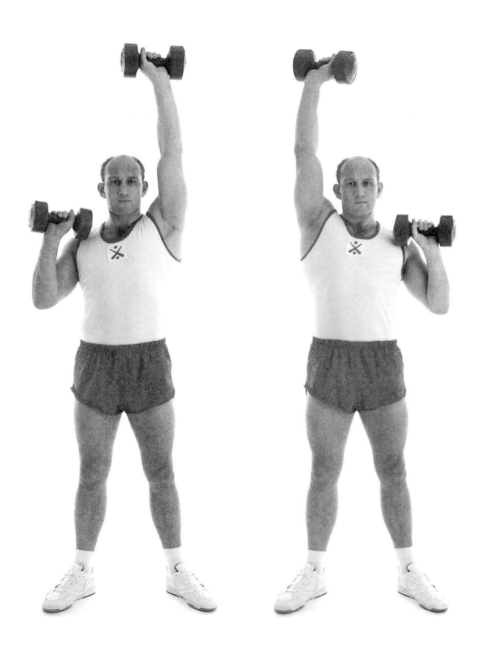

LATERAL RAISES

Main muscles used: deltoids

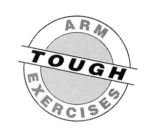

- Stand with feet shoulder-width apart, and hold a light weight or dumbbell in each hand.
- Extend arms out to sides to just over shoulder height, then lower the arms again, under control.
- Repeat.

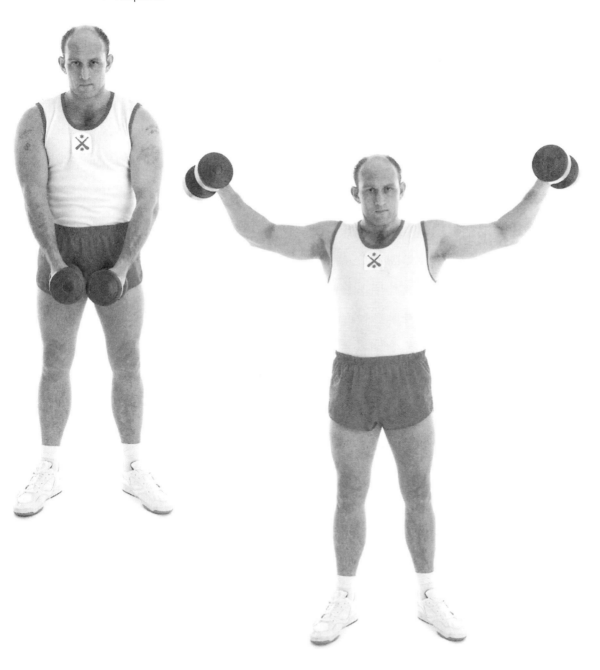

Guidlines for lifting weights

- Check all retaining collars on free weights.
- Lift weights with a straight flat back (bend your knees not your torso).
- Grip weights tightly. Keep wrists locked.
- Always place weights down under control.
- Never attempt to lift a weight that is too heavy.
- When working in pairs, get assistance from your partner.
- Stay hydrated. Wear proper footwear (cross trainers are ideal).

ARM CURLS

Main muscles used: biceps (front of upper arm)

- Stand with feet shoulder-width apart, knees soft. Hold a barbell with both hands and have arms close by your sides.
- Keeping elbows as still as possible, bend arms upwards to raise barbell in front. Slowly return to starting position.
- Repeat.

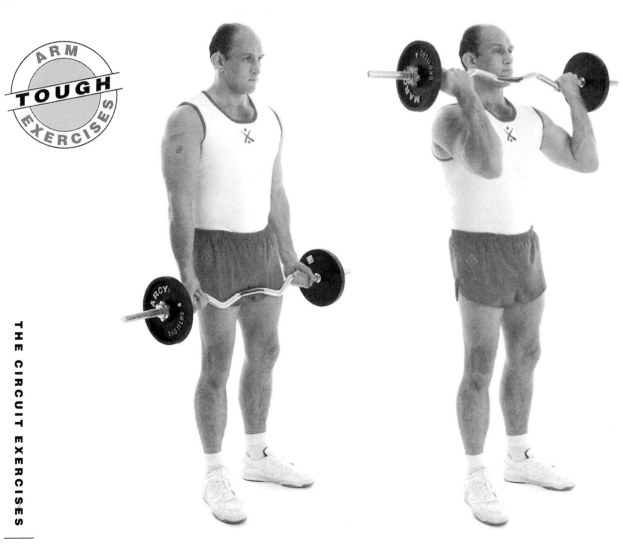

ARM TOUGH EXERCISES

PRESS-UPS

Main muscles used: triceps; deltoids; pectorals

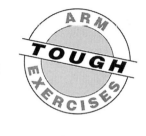

- Start face down, with hands shoulder-width apart, legs and body straight and head in line with body. Only the palms of the hands and the balls of the feet should touch the floor.
- Keeping your back straight, bend arms and lower your chest towards floor.
- Straighten arms (but do not lock elbows) and raise chest to return to starting position.
- Repeat.

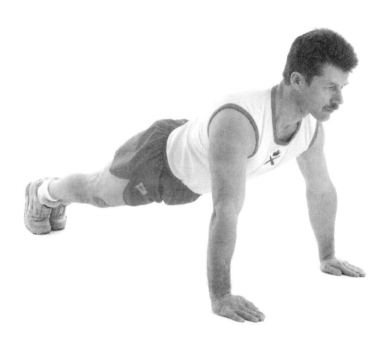

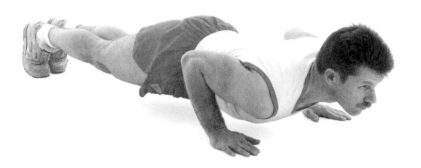

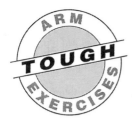

CLOSE ARM PRESS-UPS

Main muscles used: as standard press-ups

The closer together the arms in a press-up, the greater the work for the triceps (back of upper arm). The wider the arms, the greater the work for the pectorals (chest).

● Proceed as for standard press-ups but with hands placed approximately 15 cm (6 inches) apart or spread your fingers and have thumbs touching.

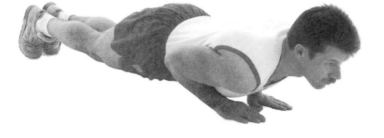

WIDE ARM PRESS-UPS

Main muscles used: as standard press-ups

● Proceed as for standard press-ups but with arms placed wider than shoulder-width apart. In the lowered position the hands should be directly under elbows.

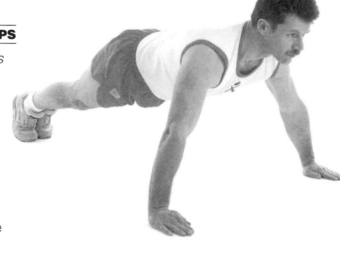

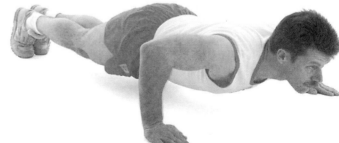

Arm Exercises: Killer

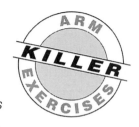

MILITARY PRESSES

Main muscles used: deltoids; upper pectorals

- Stand with feet shoulder-width apart, knees soft. Using both hands, hold a light barbell or medicine ball at chest height.
- Without locking elbows, straighten arms upwards to lift barbell or ball in the air. Bend arms to lower barbell or ball to chest, and repeat.

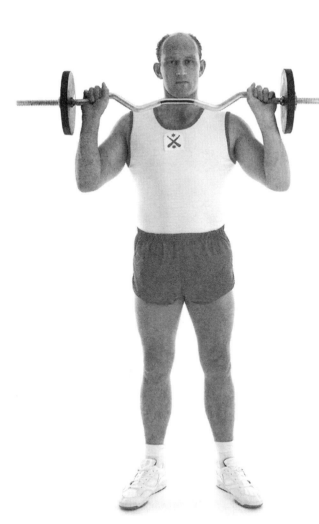

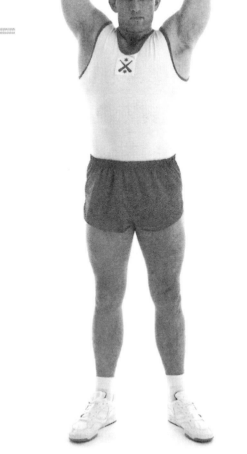

Guidlines for lifting weights

- Check all retaining collars on free weights.
- Lift weights with a straight flat back (bend your knees not your torso).
- Grip weights tightly. Keep wrists locked.
- Always place weights down under control.
- Never attempt to lift a weight that is too heavy.
- When working in pairs, get assistance from your partner.
- Stay hydrated. Wear proper footwear (cross trainers are ideal).

BEHIND THE NECK PRESSES

Main muscles used: deltoids; triceps

- Stand with feet shoulder-width apart, knees soft. Using both hands, hold a light barbell or medicine ball at the nape of the neck.
- Without locking elbows, straighten arms to push barbell or ball above head. Bend arms to return to starting position, and repeat.

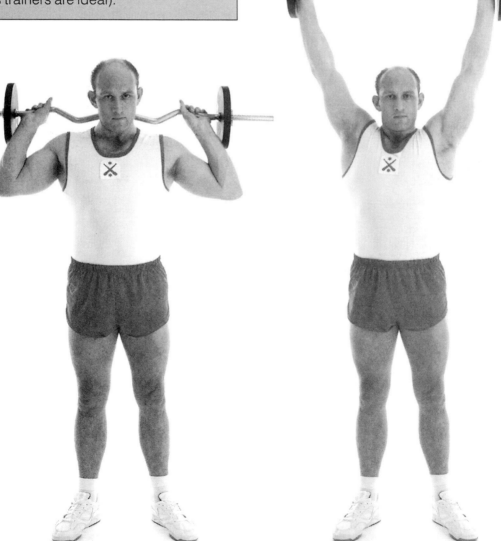

NIEDER PRESSES

Main muscles used: pectorals; deltoids

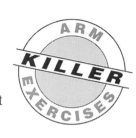

- Stand with one foot placed about 30 cm (12 inches) in front of the other, knees soft. Using both hands, hold a light barbell or medicine ball at chest height.
- Keeping barbell or ball at chest height, extend arms in front, without locking elbows. Bend arms to return to starting position, and repeat.

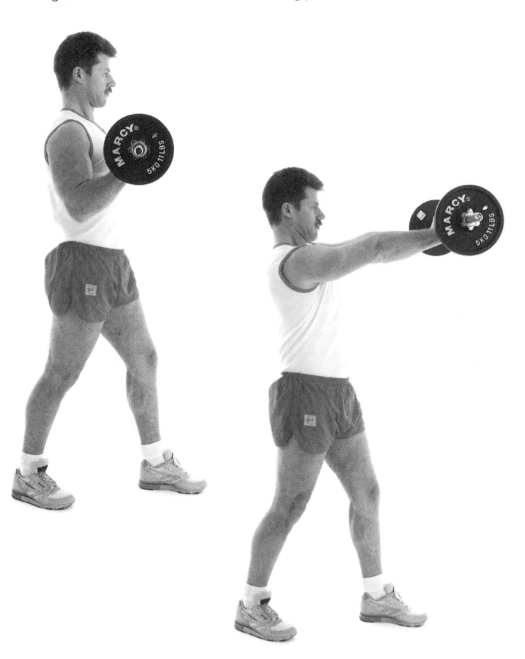

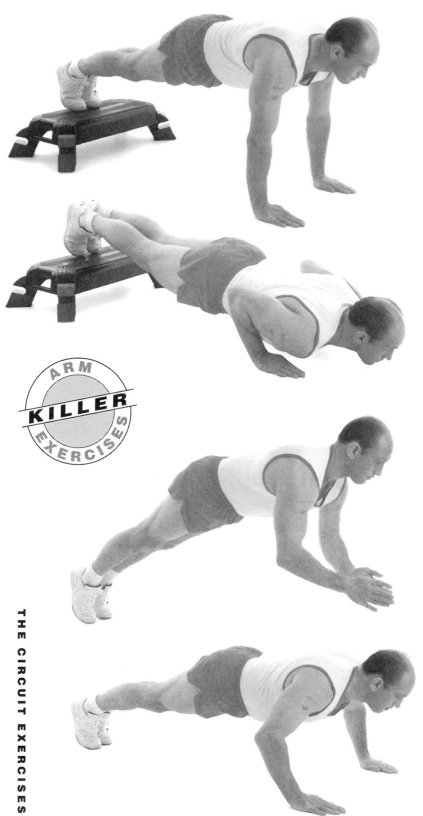

RAISED LEG PRESS-UPS

Main muscles used: triceps; deltoids; pectorals

- Start face down, with hands shoulder-width apart and balls of feet placed on raised platform or step.
- Keeping your back straight, bend arms and lower your chest towards floor.
- Straighten arms (but do not lock elbows) and raise chest to return to starting position.
- Repeat.

ARM KILLER EXERCISES

CLAP PRESS-UPS

Main muscles used: as raised leg press-ups

When you first start to practise this exercise, use a mat to cushion your hands.

- Start in the standard press-ups position with head in line with body.
- Lower your chest towards floor, then push up off floor and clap hands. Land on bent arms.
- Lift chest up to starting position, and repeat.

PULL-UPS

Main muscles used: latissimus dorsi; deltoids; triceps; biceps

Use a pull-up bar in a gym or use one from a sports shop that you can erect in a doorway at home.

- Stand and face pull-up bar and grip it tightly with both hands in either an undergrasp or overgrasp position. Arms should be straight.
- Pull yourself up off the floor with your arms until your chin is above bar. Lower yourself to floor, and repeat.

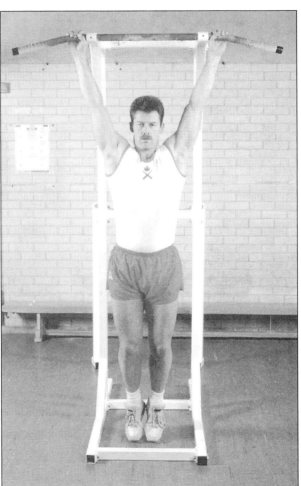

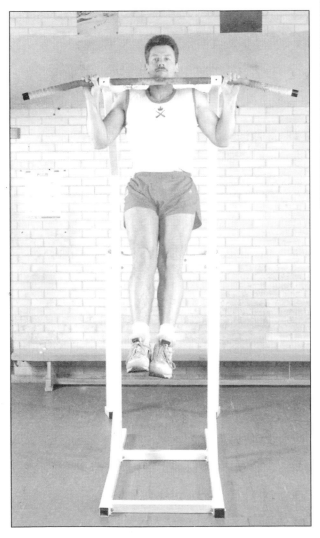

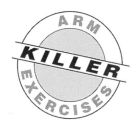

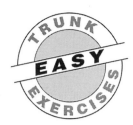

Trunk Exercises: Easy

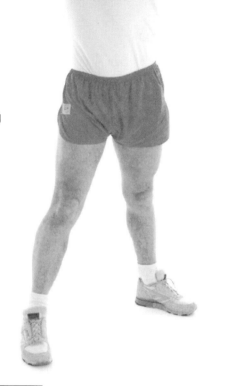

STANDING TWISTS

Main muscles used: obliques (waist)

- Stand with feet slightly wider than shoulder-width apart, knees soft. Place both hands on chest, with elbows pointing outwards.
- Slowly twist upper body to one side.
- Return through centre and twist to other side.
- Repeat, alternating sides and moving in a smooth, controlled rhythm.

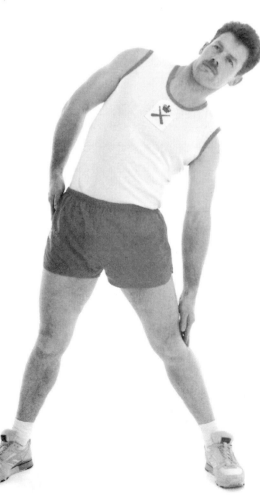

SIDE BENDS

Main muscles used: obliques

- Stand with feet slightly wider than shoulder-width apart, knees soft and arms by your sides. Keep body upright as if you were sandwiched between two plate glass windows.
- Lean directly over to one side and try to touch your knee or further down leg.
- Return up through centre and lean over to other side.
- Repeat, alternating sides and moving in a smooth, controlled rhythm.

FLOOR TOUCHES

Main muscles used: obliques; quadriceps (front of thigh); gluteals (buttocks); adductors (inner thighs)

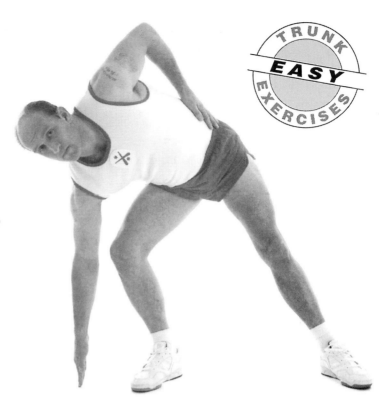

- Stand with feet slightly wider than shoulder-width apart, knees soft. Bend right knee and lean directly over to right, aiming to touch floor with right hand.
- Return through centre and repeat to other side.
- Repeat to alternate sides.

HALF-SITS

Main muscles used: abdominals (stomach)

- Lie on floor with knees bent and feet hip-width apart. Place hands on thighs.
- Slowly raise head and shoulders off floor, sliding hands up towards knees.
- Return to floor and repeat, breathing out as you come up and breathing in as you lower.

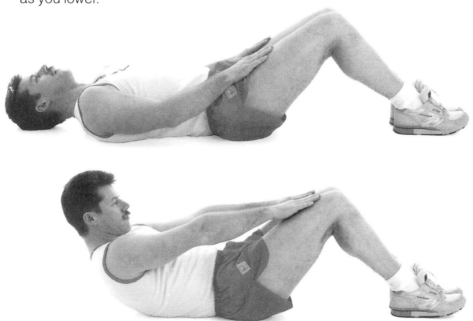

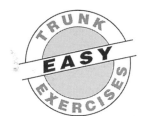

DORSAL PRESSES

Main muscles used: lower back

- Lie face down with arms bent and hands by shoulders, palms flat on floor.
- Keeping front of hips on floor, slowly raise upper body off floor.
- Return upper body to floor, and repeat.

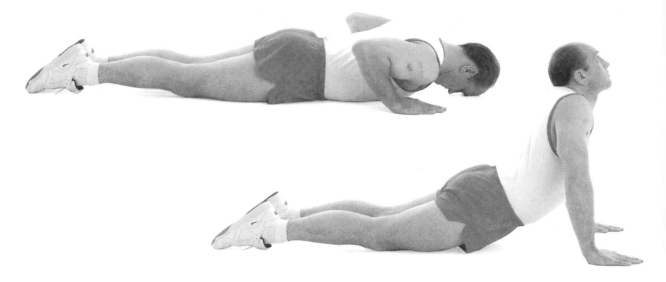

HALF DORSAL RAISES

Main muscles used: lower back

- Lie face down with hands clasped behind back.
- Keeping front of hips on floor, slowly raise upper body off floor.
- Return upper body to floor, and repeat.

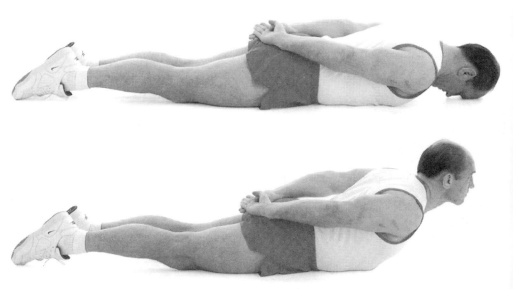

Trunk Exercises: Tough

HALF-SITS WITH TWIST

Main muscles used: obliques; abdominals

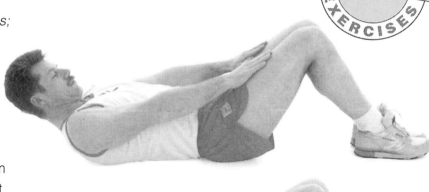

- Lie on floor with knees bent and feet hip-width apart. Place hands on thighs.
- Slowly raise head and shoulders off floor and aim left shoulder towards right knee.
- Slowly return to starting position and repeat to other side. Breathe out as you come up and breathe in as you lower.

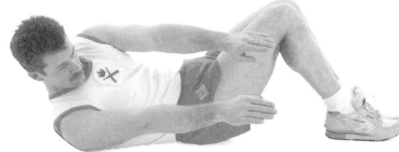

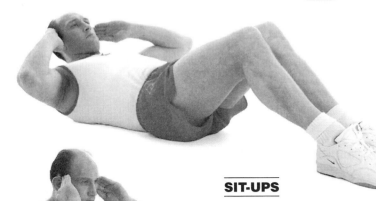

SIT-UPS

Main muscles used: abdominals; hip flexors (front of hip)

- Lie on floor with knees bent and feet hip-width apart. Place hands on temples.
- Slowly raise upper body to a sitting position.
- Slowly return to starting position and repeat, breathing out as you sit up and breathing in as you lower.

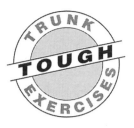

TRUNK
TOUGH
EXERCISES

SIT-UPS WITH TWIST

Main muscles used: obliques; abdominals; hip flexors

- Lie on floor with knees bent and feet hip-width apart. Place hands on temples.
- Slowly sit up and bring left elbow to right knee.
- Slowly return to starting position and repeat to other side.
- Repeat to alternate sides.

DORSAL RAISES

Main muscles used: lower back; gluteals

- Lie face down with hands clasped behind back.
- Keeping legs straight, lift head, shoulders, chest and legs off floor as high as you can.
- Return to starting position, and repeat.

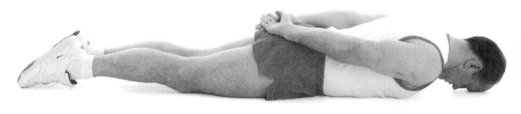

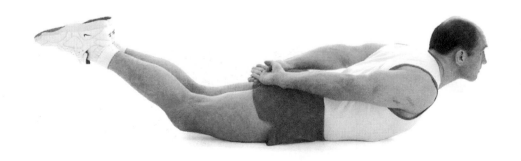

ALTERNATE DORSAL RAISES

Main muscles used: as dorsal raises

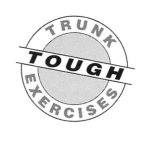

- Lie face down with arms and legs extended.
- Slowly raise left arm and right leg off floor.
- Slowly lower the arm and leg to floor, and repeat by raising right arm and left leg.
- Repeat with alternate arms/legs.

HALF V-SITS

Main muscles used: abdominals

- Lying on floor, bend knees in towards chest, then raise legs and straighten them slightly. Extend arms forwards and place hands on knees.
- Slowly raise head and shoulders off floor, taking your hands off knees and aiming hands towards feet.
- Slowly return to starting position with hands on knees.
- Repeat, breathing out as you lift and in as you lower.

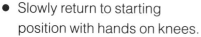

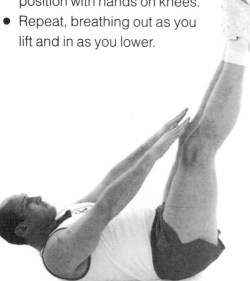

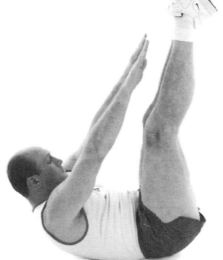

TRUNK CURLS

Main muscles used: abdominals

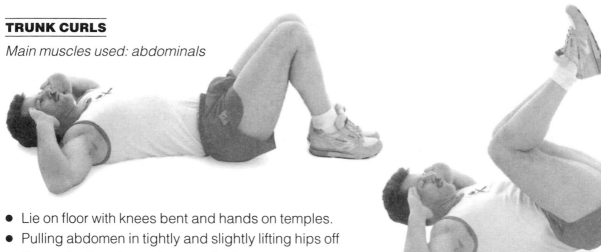

- Lie on floor with knees bent and hands on temples.
- Pulling abdomen in tightly and slightly lifting hips off floor, raise bent knees in towards chest.
- Slowly return to starting position, and repeat.

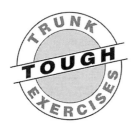

Trunk Exercises: Killer

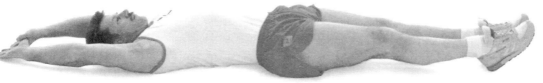

V-SITS

Main muscles used: abdominals; hip flexors

- Lie on floor with arms and legs extended.
- Keeping arms and legs straight as possible, raise head, shoulders and legs, aiming hands towards knees.
- Slowly return to starting position, and repeat. Breathe out as you raise and breathe in as you lower.

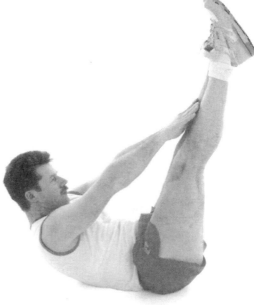

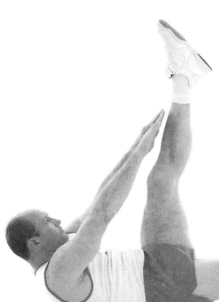

ALTERNATE V-SITS

Main muscles used: as V-sits

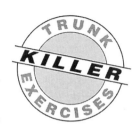

- Lie on floor with arms and legs extended.
- Keeping arms and legs as straight as possible, raise arms and one leg off floor, aiming hands towards raised leg.
- Slowly return to starting position and repeat, raising other leg. Breathe out as you raise and breathe in as you lower.
- Repeat with alternate legs.

INCLINE SIT-UPS

Main muscles used: abdominals; hip flexors

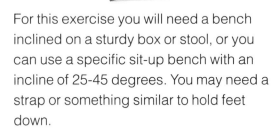

For this exercise you will need a bench inclined on a sturdy box or stool, or you can use a specific sit-up bench with an incline of 25-45 degrees. You may need a strap or something similar to hold feet down.

- Lie on bench with legs elevated. Place hands behind head.
- Slowly come up to a sitting position with knees bent.
- Slowly return to starting position, and repeat.

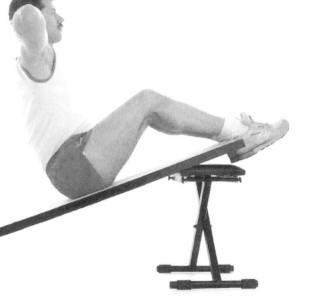

THE CIRCUIT EXERCISES

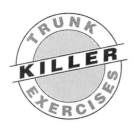

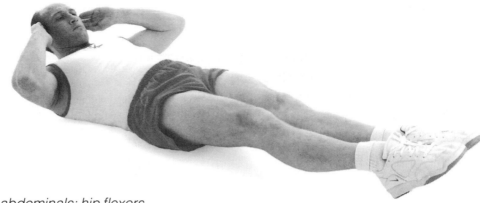

CRUNCHIES

Main muscles used: abdominals; hip flexors

- Lie down with legs extended. Place hands on temples.
- Bend then raise knees and at same time raise upper body off floor, aiming head towards knees.
- Slowly lower legs but don't let them touch the floor.
- Repeat, breathing out as you lift and breathing in as you lower.

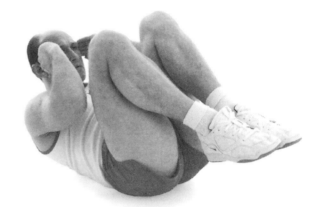

CRUNCHIES WITH TWIST

Main muscles used: abdominals; obliques; hip flexors

- Lie down with legs extended. Place hands on temples.
- Bend then raise knees and at same time raise upper body off floor, aiming left shoulder towards right knee.
- Slowly return to starting position, and repeat to other side.
- Repeat to alternate sides.

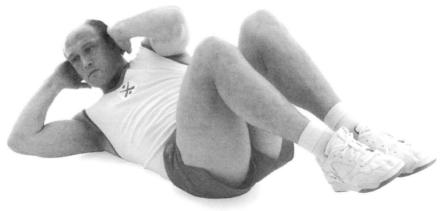

FLUTTER KICKS

Main muscles used: abdominals

- Lie on floor with arms by your sides and legs extended.
- Raise both legs a little way off floor and kick alternate legs upwards as if you were doing the leg action in a back crawl swimming stroke. Legs remain off floor for duration of reps.

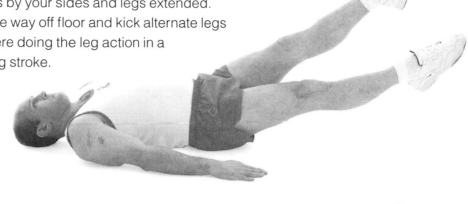

Leg Exercises: Easy

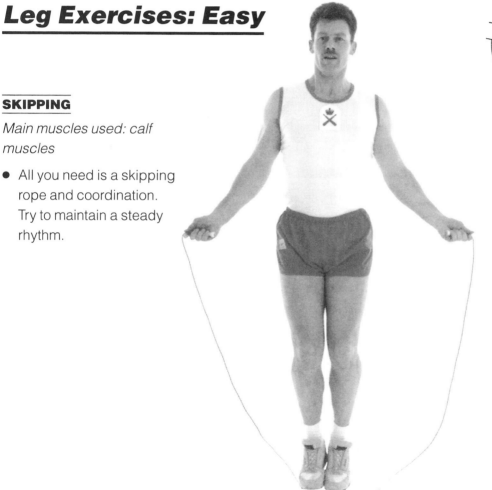

SKIPPING

Main muscles used: calf muscles

- All you need is a skipping rope and coordination. Try to maintain a steady rhythm.

LEG EASY EXERCISES

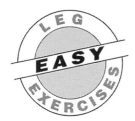

LEG EASY EXERCISES

CALF RAISES

Main muscles used: calf muscles

- Stand with heels on floor and toes raised on a plank of wood no more than 5 cm (2 inches) thick. If necessary, hold on to the back of a chair for support.
- Slowly raise heels and come up on to balls of feet.
- Lower heels back to floor, and repeat.

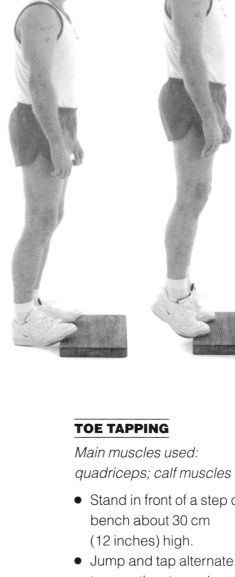

TOE TAPPING

Main muscles used: quadriceps; calf muscles

- Stand in front of a step or bench about 30 cm (12 inches) high.
- Jump and tap alternate toes on the step or bench. Try to get a momentum going.

FORWARD LUNGES

Main muscles used: quadriceps; hamstrings (back of thigh); hip flexors; gluteals

- Stand upright with knees soft and hands on hips.
- Keeping back straight, extend one leg forwards and go down into lunge position with both knees bent and upper body centred between legs. Front knee should be directly above ankle.
- Push up to return to starting position, and repeat with other leg. Do an equal number of reps on each leg.

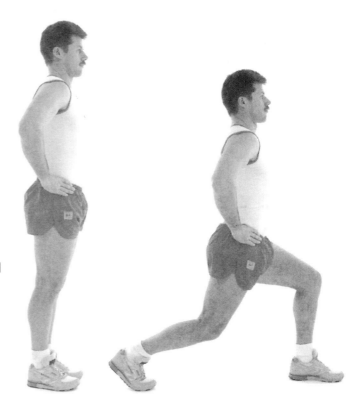

Leg Exercises: Tough

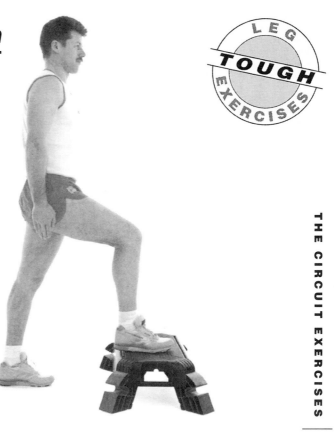

STEP-UPS

Main muscles used: quadriceps; calf muscles

- Stand in front of a step or bench between 20 and 35 cm (8 and 14 inches) high (no higher).
- Step up with right foot, making sure you place whole of foot on step.
- Step up with left foot.
- Step down with right foot, then follow with left foot, and repeat.
- Repeat, this time leading with left leg, making sure you do an equal number of reps on each leg.

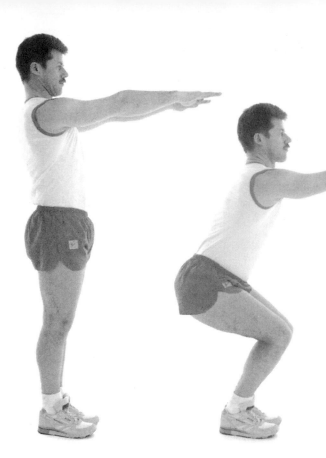

SQUATS

Main muscles used: quadriceps; gluteals; lower back

- Stand upright with knees soft, and arms extended in front.

- Keeping your back straight, slowly bend knees and push your backside backwards as if about to sit in a chair, but don't let backside go below line of knees.
- Slowly return to starting position, and repeat.

SQUAT THRUSTS

Main muscles used: quadriceps; hip flexors; deltoids (statically)

- Start in the standard press-ups position with arms below shoulders, legs outstretched, chest off floor and back straight.
- Jump both legs forward to crouch position so that knees are in line with elbows.
- Jump legs back to starting position and repeat, keeping on balls of feet throughout.

LEG
TOUGH
EXERCISES

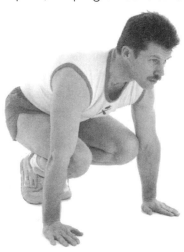

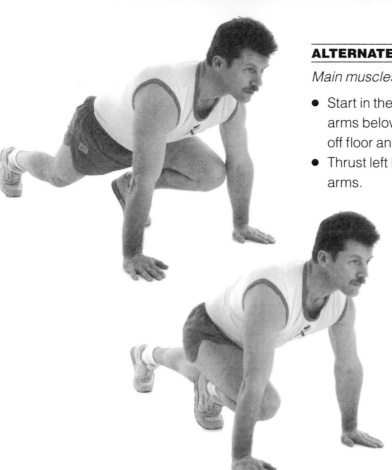

ALTERNATE SQUAT THRUSTS

Main muscles used: as squat thrusts

- Start in the standard press-ups position with arms below shoulders, legs outstretched, chest off floor and back straight.
- Thrust left leg forwards until knee is through arms.
- Bring left leg back and thrust right leg forwards.
- Continue to thrust alternate legs forwards at speed, remaining on balls of feet throughout.

SPLIT JUMPS

Main muscles used: quadriceps; calf muscles; hamstrings

- Go down into a semi-crouch position with one leg forwards, and prepare to jump.
- Jump up into air, with one leg forwards and one back.
- Land on bended knees and return to semi-crouch position to get ready for next jump.
- Jump up into air again and switch position of legs.
- Repeat split jumps, alternating legs.

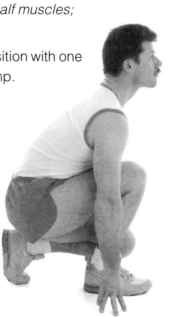

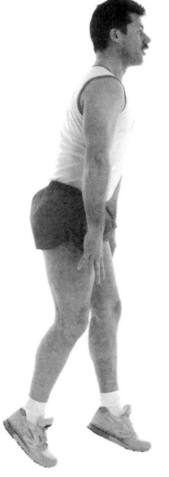

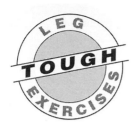

STRIDE JUMPS

Main muscles used: quadriceps; calf muscles

- Stand upright with feet together, knees soft, and arms by your sides.
- Jump legs wide apart, extending arms outwards and upwards. Do not aim to jump too high.
- Land on bent knees, and repeat.

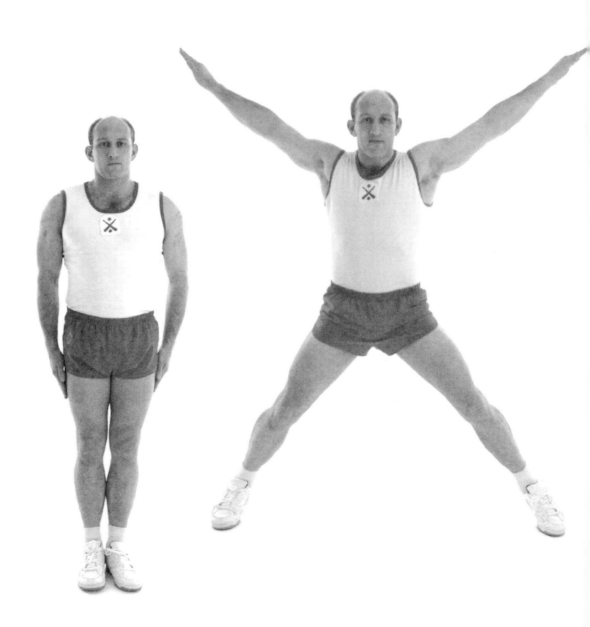

STAR JUMPS

Main muscles used: quadriceps; calf muscles; hamstrings

- Stand upright with feet together, knees soft and arms by your sides.
- Go down into the crouch position with hands on floor and arms inside knees.
- Jump as high as you can with arms and legs outstretched.
- Land on bent knees and go down into crouch position.
- Repeat.

LEG TOUGH EXERCISES

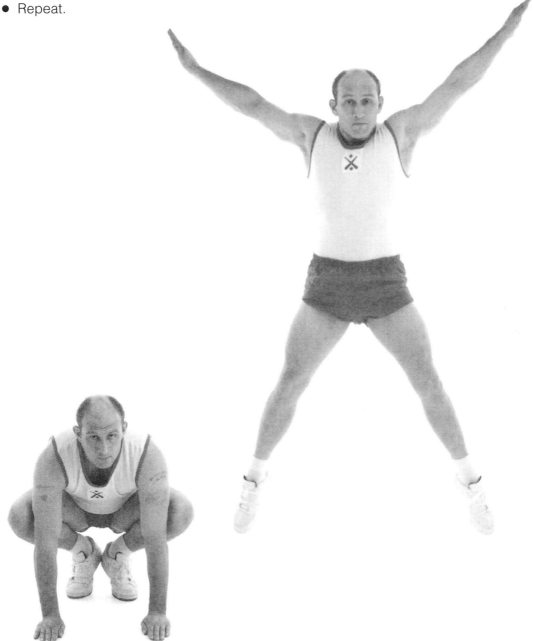

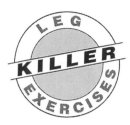

Leg Exercises: Killer

TUCK JUMPS

Main muscles used: quadriceps; calf muscles

- Stand with feet together, knees soft, and arms by your sides.
- Jump as high as you can, aiming knees towards chest. (Do not bring chest down to meet knees.)
- Land on bent knees, and repeat.

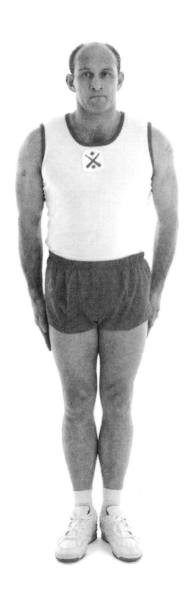
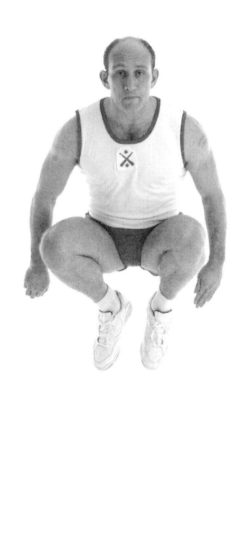

SERGEANT JUMPS

Main muscles used: hamstrings; gluteals; calf muscles;

This exercise needs to be performed near a wall. Place a mark on the wall about 2.4-2.7 metres (8-9 ft) high.

- Stand near wall and go down into crouch position.
- Jump up and aim to touch mark on wall. Make sure you land on bent knees.
- Repeat.

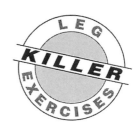

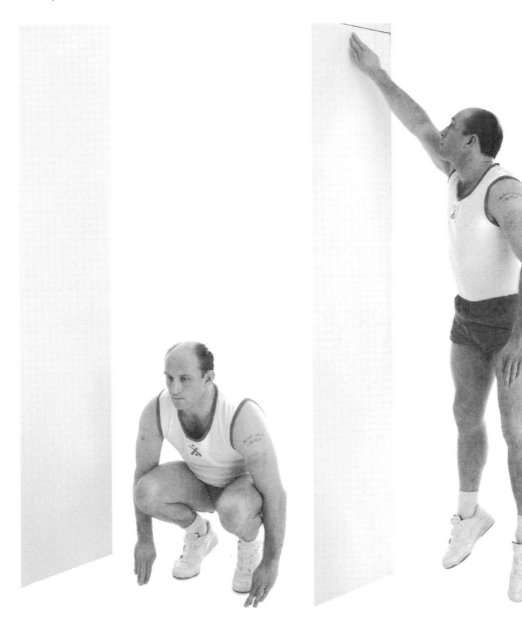

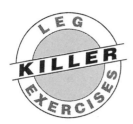

BUM JUMPS

Main muscles used: quadriceps; calf muscles; hamstrings

- Stand upright on top of a bench, knees soft and arms by your sides.
- Jump feet apart to either side of bench and bring backside down towards, but do not touch, bench.
- Jump up on to bench, and repeat.

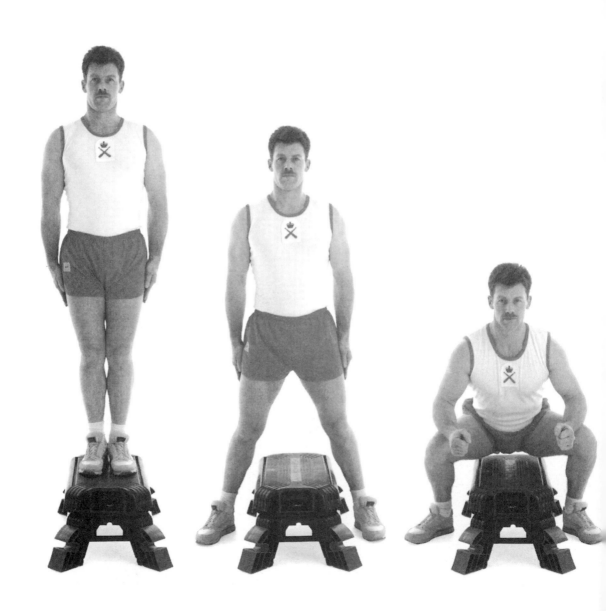

LATERAL JUMPS

Main muscles used: quadriceps; hamstrings; calf muscles

Use a bench or place a bar across two Jerry cans or boxes about 60 cm (2 ft) high.

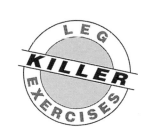

- Stand sideways on to the bench or bar, with feet together, knees soft.
- Jump sideways over the bar and immediately jump back over it again.
- Continue jumping like this. If you tire, you can do a double bounce on each side.

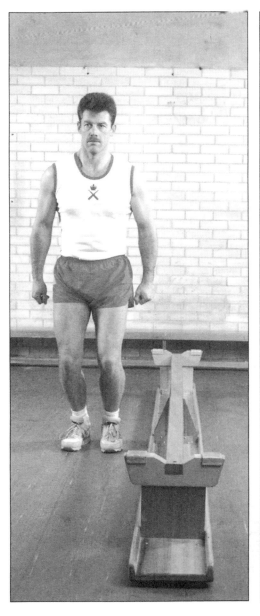
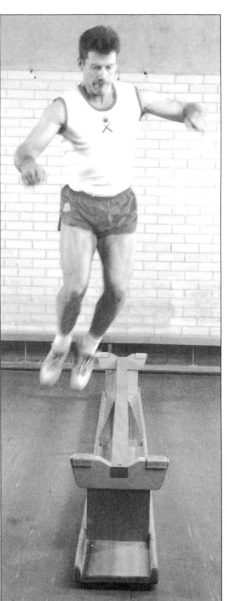

BOX JUMPS

Main muscles used:
quadriceps; calf muscles;
hamstrings

Line up three boxes, leaving an equal distance between each. The first should be approximately 60 cm (2 ft) high, the second 45 cm (18 inches), and the third 30 cm (12 inches).

- Stand with feet together, knees soft, in front of the first box. Bend knees and take off with a two-footed jump to land in front of second box. Immediately take off again to jump over the second box, then the third.
- Run back to starting position and repeat.

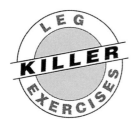

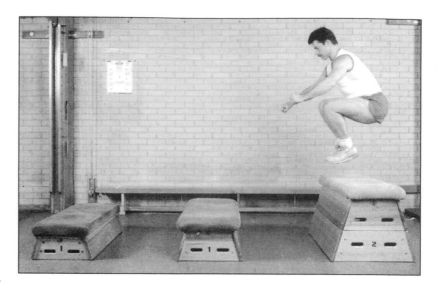

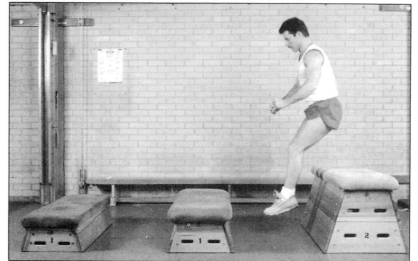

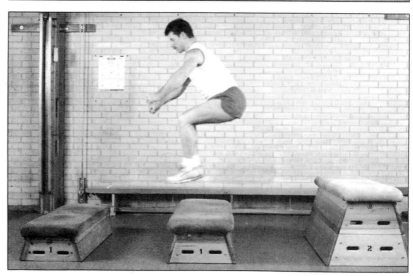

BURPEES (KILLER+)

Main muscles used: majority of muscles in body

1 Stand upright, with feet together and knees soft.
2 Go down into crouch position with hands on floor.
3 Jump legs backwards to press-ups position with chest off floor.
4 Jump legs forwards to crouch position.
5 Stand upright again.
● Repeat in a fluid motion, making sure you return to the standing position at the end of each rep.

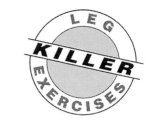

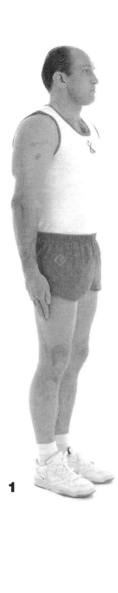

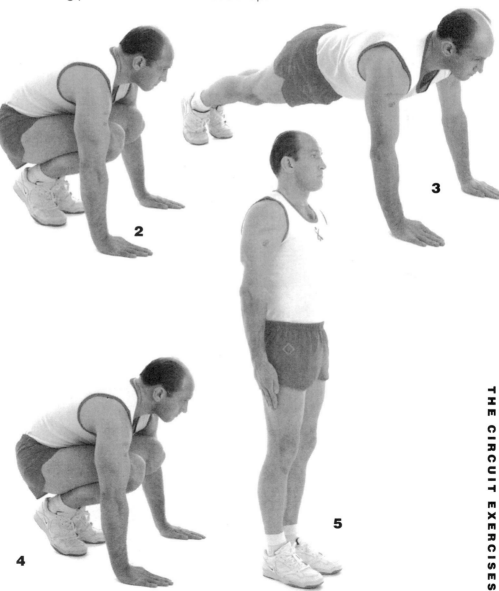

1

2

3

4

5

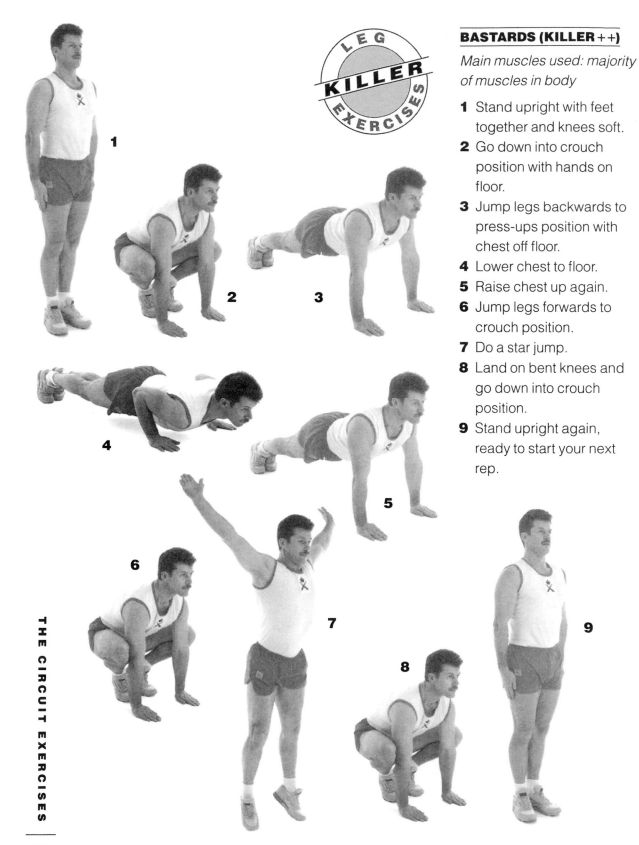

LEG KILLER EXERCISES

BASTARDS (KILLER++)

Main muscles used: majority of muscles in body

1 Stand upright with feet together and knees soft.
2 Go down into crouch position with hands on floor.
3 Jump legs backwards to press-ups position with chest off floor.
4 Lower chest to floor.
5 Raise chest up again.
6 Jump legs forwards to crouch position.
7 Do a star jump.
8 Land on bent knees and go down into crouch position.
9 Stand upright again, ready to start your next rep.

The Nod Circuit Programme

OK. Now you know the nitty-gritty about what you should eat, warming up, stretching, mobilising and cooling down, it's time to get to the meat – grilled chicken breast without skin – and potatoes (baked) of the book.

The first eight weeks – the Nod Circuit Programme – are designed to take an unfit man to an overall level of physical fitness where he is capable of taking on and beating the Beast. Week 1 involves a beginner's circuit. It consist of seven exercises and is carried out using the Timed Circuit procedure. We use these first exercises because they are simple to perform and use all the major muscle groups. Get them right and you are well on the way.

WEEK ONE

CIRCUITS THIS WEEK: 3

Day 1: Timed Circuit

Number of circuits: 2-3 depending on level
    of fitness. Try two and see how you feel.
Exercise time: 15 seconds per exercise
Rest between exercises: 10 seconds
Rest between circuits: 1 minute
Exercises per circuit: 7

Circuit Exercises

1 **HALF-SITS**
2 **DORSAL RAISES**
3 **PRESS-UPS**
4 **SQUAT THRUSTS**
5 **SIT-UPS**
6 **DIPS**
7 **STEP-UPS**

Important

Keep a note of which circuits you do each day. During the programme, you will be instructed to repeat the exercises you do on a particular day and unless you've got a fantastic memory you will forget what to do when – so write everything down!

Day 2: Complete Rest

Take it easy, but don't forget to do all those stretching and mobilisation exercises. It is important to sleep well on rest days.

Day 3: Timed Circuit

As Day 1.

Day 4: Complete Rest

Take it easy, but don't forget to do all those stretching and mobilisation exercises.

Day 5: Complete Rest

Take it easy, but don't forget to do all those stretching and mobilisation exercises.

Day 6: Timed Circuit

As Days 1 and 3.

If by the third and final circuit of the week you are feeling confident, you may add variety by changing the format to that of a repetition circuit (so instead of doing each exercise for 15 seconds you can do a set number of reps). By this time you will know how many reps you can perform in the 15 seconds. Now add a further two reps to each exercise and perform the exercise much more slowly. While it sounds simple this will really challenge you. Work in your full range of movement thus making each exercise slightly harder still. On no account add more than two additional reps.

This is the first week so don't blow it by risking overtraining and injury. It's going to get harder. That's a promise. And a warning.

Day 7: Complete Rest

Take it easy, but don't forget to do all those stretching and mobilisation exercises.

> **In all circuits you should always use the ATL approach. This means doing Arm, Trunk (including one lower back or dorsal exercise) and Leg exercises in any order.**

WEEK TWO

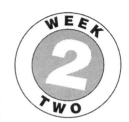

CIRCUITS THIS WEEK: 4

Yesterday you were probably a little stiff from the first week's activities. If you *are* stiff don't take the couch-potato option and slob out on the sofa with six pints of lager and a video. First do your stretching and mobilisation routine slowly and carefully. Hold the stretches where you can feel something happening for an extra 5 seconds. Now you can slob out … but you've got to lose the lager. **The alcohol ban is still in operation**.

Week 2 is going to be tough. It is a crucial point in the Nod Circuit Programme. It's also time to add a little variety. At the end of the week you will be taking a Test, which will also be taken at the end of Weeks 5 and 8. This Test will be a benchmark by which you can measure your level of fitness – and your commitment. Secondly we are bringing in the concept of Active Rest, twice a week.

First we are going to increase the amount of exercises in each circuit from seven up to nine. These nine exercises are our Core Exercises, the basic components of physical fitness. Learn them and learn them properly so that by the end of this week they are second nature to you.

> ### Motivation Tip
>
> - Before you start training, weigh yourself wearing just exercise shorts. Now measure your vital statistics – chest, waist, biceps, thighs, and stomach. Make a note of these and put it away for four weeks.

Day 1: The Test Circuit

Week 2 starts with a bang. Welcome to the Test Circuit, which you are going to get to know very well. Either write down or photocopy the chart on the next pages and then follow the instructions below.

Instructions for Day 1

1 After your warm-up, perform each exercise (see next pages) correctly, and as fast as possible. Then rest for 1 minute while you note in the Test Reps column the amount of repetitions you achieved. Now move on to the next exercise and repeat the process until you have completed all nine, noting your score each time.

2 In the Training Reps column, write half your original score, marking down if it was an odd number originally eg Half-sits Test Reps = 19, Training Reps: 9; Dorsal raises Test Reps = 17, Training Reps = 8. You will be grateful for this small mercy within the next 5 minutes!

3 You have learnt both individual exercises and their sequence. Now comes the hard part – the Test Circuit.

4 Start the stop watch and GO. You must carry out the required number of repetitions of the nine exercises without pausing between each exercise. Each individual circuit must be performed three times through without rest. Because the training reps are half of the test reps you will be able to give it your best shot and really have a go at the test.

5 At the end, make a note of the time you took. Now calculate 75 per cent of this to find your Target Time. For instance if it took 12 minutes to complete all three circuits (and a further 3 minutes to stop gasping for air) your Target Time is now 9 minutes.

Right now that probably looks impossible. But as Donald Sutherland says in *Kelly's Heroes* 'stop making with those negative waves'. You have already achieved more than you think. Remember all those Test Reps? Well, they took it out of your body. Next time you don't have to do them. Instead you do a warm-up followed by an all-out assault on that Target Time. We are not completely inhuman, but at the end of Weeks 5 and 8 the Target Time will be two-thirds of the Test Time. Isn't that something to look forward to?

Exercises	Test Time	Test Reps	Training Reps (half your Test Reps score)
HALF-SITS	20 secs	_____	_____
DORSAL RAISES	20 secs	_____	_____
PRESS-UPS	20 secs	_____	_____
SQUAT THRUSTS	20 secs	_____	_____

Exercises		Test Time	Test Reps	Training Reps (half your Test Reps score)
SIT-UPS		20 secs	_____	_____
DIPS		20 secs	_____	_____
STEP-UPS		20 secs	_____	_____
SIDE BENDS		20 secs	_____	_____
CRUNCHIES		20 secs	_____	_____

Test Time _____ **Actual Time** _____ **Target Time** _____

Important note

If you fail to complete the Test Circuit in the Target Time don't be downhearted. All it means is that you are not quite ready to go on to Week 3. Tomorrow take a day of Complete Rest. Then simply repeat Week 2. Next time you should waltz through.

Day 2: Active Rest

There is a limit to the amount of circuit exercises you can and should do. Too much leads to overexertion, muscle strains and in severe cases long-term injury. Also, too much repetition is boring – Active Rest provides a variation. Don't forget to warm up with gentle stretching and mobilisation exercises.

On Active Rest days you don't have to try to beat a time or increase the distance covered. However, as the programme progresses most people will naturally try to beat previous performances. Do remember these are meant to be **rest** days when you are carrying out a different activity at a lower intensity. It is vital that you vary the activity. Don't stick to just jogging, walking or cycling. Today, go for a brisk 30-minute **WALK** (walking helps to diminish the sensation of stiffness which always comes after intensive training).

Day 3: Timed Circuit

Number of circuits: 3 times through
Exercise time: 15 seconds per exercise
Rest between exercises: 10 seconds
Rest between circuits: 1 minute
Exercises per circuit: 9

You take the same nine Core Exercises you practised on Day 1, but here you do a timed circuit like Week 1.

Day 4: Complete Rest

Do only stretching exercises, and go to bed early.

Day 5: Timed Circuit

As Day 3.

Day 6: Active Rest

Go for an easy 15-20 minute swim or jog at a consistent speed or a 20-30 minute cycle in easy gears.

Day 7: Test Circuit

Warm up carefully. Go through each of the Core Exercises slowly (do 2-3 repetitions). After this, double-check you know the order they have to be done in, and that the bench for the dips and the step-ups is in a position where it will not get in the way of any other exercise.

Take 15 seconds to breathe deeply. Now, go for it.

WEEK THREE

CIRCUITS THIS WEEK: 3

Day 1: Complete Rest

Day 2: Timed Circuit

Number of circuits: 3 times through
Exercise time: 15 seconds per exercise
Rest between exercises: 10 seconds
Rest between circuits: 1 minute
Exercises per circuit: 9

Motivation Tip

Always stay hydrated. Get into the habit of drinking water – at least 2 litres a day. Keep a large bottle of mineral water to hand and sip from it constantly. Coffee and tea, like booze, are diuretics – they make you urinate. The easiest way to check for dehydration is to look at the colour of your urine. The yellower your pee the more dehydrated you are. It can take over two hours to hydrate the body fully.

Circuit 1

1 PRESS-UPS
2 TRUNK CURLS
3 ALTERNATE LEG
  SQUAT THRUSTS
4 ARM CURLS
5 SIT-UPS
6 HALF DORSAL RAISES
7 DIPS
8 HALF-SITS
9 STRIDE JUMPS

Circuit 2

1 ARM PUNCHES
2 CRUNCHIES
3 STEP-UPS
4 DIPS
5 HALF-SITS
6 SQUAT THRUSTS
7 DORSAL PRESSES
8 SIT-UPS
9 SPLIT JUMPS

You may choose any one of these four circuits, which are similar in intensity and muscular endurance. However, to avoid boredom and prevent cheating you should do all the circuits over the next two weeks.

Circuit 3

1 DIPS
2 HALF-SITS
3 TOE TAPPING
4 ARM CURLS
5 SIT-UPS WITH TWIST
6 STEP-UPS OR SQUATS
7 DORSAL PRESSES
8 CRUNCHIES
9 TUCK JUMPS

Circuit 4

1 MILITARY PRESSES
2 CRUNCHIES
3 STEP-UPS
4 DORSAL RAISES
5 SIT-UPS
6 STRIDE JUMPS
7 DIPS
8 SIT-UPS WITH TWIST
9 SQUAT THRUSTS

Day 3: Active Rest

Activity	Time in minutes	Pace
Walk	15-20	Brisk

If you are reasonably fit you may wish to jog instead. Only you know your level of ability. If you do want to jog, walk briskly for the first 5 minutes, jog for 10-15 minutes, then cool down by walking for another 5 minutes. Don't forget to warm up with gentle stretching and mobilisation exercises.

Day 4: Timed Circuit

As Day 2.

Day 5: Complete Rest

Take it easy, but don't forget to stretch and mobilise.

Day 6: Timed Circuit

This is the same format as Days 2 and 4 but you should now switch to a different set of circuit exercises.

Day 7: Active Rest

Activity	Time in minutes	Pace	Remarks
Cycling	30-40	Easy	Use easy gears

WEEK FOUR

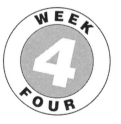

CIRCUITS THIS WEEK: 3

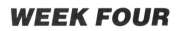

Day 1: Timed Circuit

Do the same circuit as you did on Day 6 last week.

Day 2: Active Rest

Activity	Time in minutes	Pace	Remarks
Swimming	20-25	Easy	Straight swim

Day 3: Timed Circuit

This is the same format as Day 1, but switch to another set of circuit exercises.

Day 4: Complete Rest

Take it easy, but don't forget to stretch and mobilise.

Day 5: Active Rest

Activity	Time in minutes	Pace	Remarks
Walk/jog	15-20	Brisk	Jog a little

Day 6: Timed Circuit

As Day 3 but as you've had a couple of days' resting you might want to be brave and tackle the final choice of circuit.

Day 7: Complete Rest

Don't forget to do all those stretching and mobilisation exercises.

WEEK FIVE

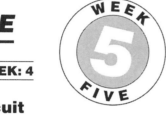

CIRCUITS THIS WEEK: 4

Day 1: Test Circuit

Remember the Test Circuit you did in Week 2? It's time to do it again. Go through the testing procedure exactly as you did last time (see pages 85-87), do the same exercises and make notes of the number of reps and the time you take to complete. The bad news is that your Target Time is now two-thirds of the Test Time.

Day 2: Complete Rest

Take it easy, but don't forget to stretch and mobilise.

Day 3: Timed Circuit

Number of circuits: 3 times through
Exercise time: 15 seconds per exercise for first two circuits,
    10 seconds per exercise for third circuit
Rest between exercises: 10 seconds
Rest between circuits: 1 minute first and second circuits,
    none between second and third circuits
Exercises per circuit: 10 (see next page)

You may choose either of the following circuits but you will end up doing both.

Circuit 1

1 MILITARY PRESSES
2 HALF-SITS
3 SQUAT THRUSTS
4 ARM CURLS
5 V-SITS
6 STRIDE JUMPS
7 PRESS-UPS
8 SIT-UPS WITH TWIST
9 TUCK JUMPS
10 DORSAL RAISES

Circuit 2

1 SQUAT THRUSTS
2 DIPS
3 CRUNCHIES
4 STEP-UPS
5 ARM CURLS
6 V-SITS
7 ALTERNATE SQUAT
   THRUSTS
8 PRESS-UPS
9 HALF-SITS
10 DORSAL PRESSES

Day 4: Active Rest

Activity	Time in minutes	Pace	Remarks
Walk/jog	20-25	Easy	Jog for about half the time

Day 5: Timed Circuit

As Day 3. You might prefer to alternate the circuits and do Circuit 2 today, Circuit 1 next time and so on. It's up to you.

Day 6: Active Rest

Activity	Time in minutes	Pace	Remarks
Cycling	30-40	Fartlek*	Go at your own pace

* *Fartlek* is Swedish for Speed Play. Basically you cycle, swim, run as you please, but by throwing in different spontaneous choices you keep yourself alert.

   For example when cycling you should vary the pace: decide to bike really fast the first 400 metres of your route, or take a hill incline at full speed. If running you can play tag with every other lamp post, even play jump the lines on the pavement stones like a kid. It may seem strange to passers-by but it will put a smile on your face as it builds up speed and strength.

Day 7: Test Circuit

Warm up carefully. Although your body should be used to all the Core Exercises by now, make sure you go through each one slowly. Do 2-3 repetitions making sure that all the right muscles are ready to go. When you have been through all the exercises, double-check you know the order they have to be done in, and that the bench for the dips and the step-ups is in a position where it will not get in the way of any other exercise.

Take 15 seconds to breathe deeply. Now, go for it.

If you fail to complete the Test Circuit in the Target Time don't be downhearted. All it means is that you are not quite ready to go on to Week 6. Tomorrow take a day of Complete Rest. After that simply repeat Week 5. Next time you should waltz through the Test.

WEEK SIX

CIRCUITS THIS WEEK: 4

Day 1: Timed Circuit

Number of circuits: 3 times through
Exercise time: 15 seconds per exercise
    first two circuits, 10 seconds per exercise for the third circuit
Rest between exercises: none
Rest between circuits: 1 minute between first and second circuits, none
    between second and third circuits
Exercises per circuit: 10

Choose your circuit from the two that you did in week 5.

Day 2: Complete Rest

Take it easy, but don't forget to do all those stretching and mobilisation exercises.

Day 3: Timed Circuit

It's your choice of circuit today.

> **The Pull-up** is a great exercise for the upper back, although in hauling up your whole body weight it's always the arms that give out first. From Week 5 if you have access to a pull-up bar, you may substitute pull-ups for *any* arm exercise.

> **It's getting hard now! The exercises have got slightly tougher, more have been added and the rest period is being reduced.**

Day 4: Active Rest

Activity	Time in minutes	Pace	Remarks
Swimming	20-25	Fartlek	Increase pace as you please

Day 5: Timed Circuit

It's your choice of circuit today.

Day 6: Active Rest

Activity	Time in minutes	Pace	Remarks
Walk/jog	20-25	Easy	Jog about half the time

Day 7: Timed Circuit

Do the circuit you didn't do on Day 5.

WEEK SEVEN

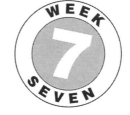

CIRCUITS PER WEEK: 4

Day 1: Active Rest

Activity	Time in minutes	Pace	Remarks
Jogging	20	Steady	Enjoy it

Day 2: Timed Circuit

Number of circuits: 3 times through
Exercise time: 15 seconds per exercise on the first circuit, 15 seconds per exercise on the second, 10 seconds per exercise on the third
Rest between exercises: None
Rest between circuits: 1 minute between first and second circuits, none between second and third circuits
Exercises per circuit: 12

You may choose either of the circuits on offer but you will end up doing both.

Don't kid yourself, this is tough! There is a purpose to our cruelty because you have not one but *two* tough tests coming up. Listen to your body very carefully over the next two weeks. If you overtrain and exhaust yourself you can kiss goodbye to passing the Test. While we suggest one Complete Rest day and two Active Rest days each week, you might wish to change the emphasis to give your body a longer time to recover. Listen to your body.

Day 3: Complete Rest

Take it easy, but don't forget to stretch and mobilise.

Day 4: Timed Circuit

Choose a different circuit from Day 2.

Day 5: Timed Circuit

Choose a different circuit from Day 4.

Day 6: Active Rest

Activity	Time in minutes	Pace	Remarks
Cycling	30-40	Steady	Do 5-10 minutes at gentle pace (warm-up), for 20-25 minutes increase pace, then 5 minutes gentle pace (cool-down). Stretch for 10 minutes afterwards concentrating on the legs.

Day 7: Test Circuit

Remember the Test Circuit you did in Weeks 2 and 5? It's time to do it again. Go through the testing procedure exactly as you did last time (see pages 85-87). Do the same exercises, make notes of the number of reps and the time you take to complete. Your Target Time is still two-thirds of the Test Time.

Circuit 1

1 WIDE ARM PRESS-UPS
2 CRUNCHIES
3 TUCK JUMPS
4 DIPS
5 V-SITS
6 STRIDE JUMPS
7 PRESS-UPS
8 DORSAL RAISES
9 SQUAT THRUSTS
10 ARM CURLS
11 HALF-SITS
12 BURPEES

Circuit 2

1 ARM CURLS
2 DORSAL PRESSES
3 BURPEES
4 CLOSE ARM PRESS-UPS
5 V-SITS
6 STAR JUMPS
7 WIDE ARM PRESS-UPS
8 SIT-UPS WITH TWIST
9 STEP-UPS OR SQUATS
10 CLAP PRESS-UPS
11 SIT-UPS
12 ALTERNATE SQUAT THRUSTS

Measure and note your vital statistics again. Compare what you find with your measurements before you started this programme. There should be a significant improvement.

WEEK EIGHT

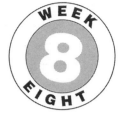

CIRCUITS PER WEEK: 4

Day 1: Timed Circuit

Number of circuits: 3 times through
Exercise time: 15 seconds per exercise first circuit, 10 seconds per exercise second circuit, 15 seconds per exercise third circuit
Rest between exercises: None
Rest between circuits: None – straight through 3 times
Exercises per circuit: 12

Day 2: Complete Rest

Take it easy, but don't forget to stretch and mobilise.

Day 3: Timed Circuit

Your choice of circuit.

Day 4: Active Rest

Activity	Time in minutes	Pace	Remarks
Swimming	20-30	Steady	Do a 5-10 minute gentle swim (warm-up), for 20-25 minutes increase pace, then 5 minutes gentle swim (cool-down)

Day 5: Timed Circuit

Your choice of circuit.

Day 6: Active Rest

Activity	Time in minutes	Pace	Remarks
Jogging	20	Steady	Increase pace to suit own ability

Day 7: Test Circuit

Warm up carefully. Although your body should be used to all the Core Exercises by now, make sure you go through each one slowly. Do 2-3 repetitions to make sure that all the right muscles are ready to go. When you have been through all the exercises, double-check you know the order they have to be done in, and that the bench for the dips and the step-ups is in a position where it will not get in the way of any other exercise.

Take 15 seconds to breathe deeply. Now, go for it.

If you fail to complete the Test Circuit in the Target Time don't be downhearted. All it means is that you are not quite ready to go on to tackle the Beast. Tomorrow take a day of Complete Rest. After that simply repeat Week 8. Next time you are should waltz through the Test.

BEAST WEEK

So, after eight weeks you've finished the Nod Circuit Programme and now you think you're ready for bigger and better things. However just because you've managed to scrape inside your Target Time on the Week 8 Test does not mean you're fit. If you thought the last two weeks were tough, wait till you tackle the Beast. Nobody's ready until they have conquered the Beast.

Day 1: Complete Rest

You'll need it! Choose which Beast you want to tackle. Now sit down and contemplate the horror in store.

Day 2: Active Rest

Go for a good 30-minute jog or long cycle ride. During this run/ride you should be scouting the perfect lair for the Beast. The Beast can be carried out inside but by using grass and park benches it gives a bit of variety, plenty of fresh air – and the possibility of an audience.

If you want to do the simple Beast, find a park bench with a nice stretch of grass next to it, where you can jog uninterrupted by paths, dog toilets and roller-bladers for 10 seconds. The grass area needs to be about 20-30 metres long and can be flat or hilly but at the end of your short jog the ground must be flat. For the Running Beast you will need a much larger expanse of open ground and might want to consider using a running track.

Take your time to find the right spot because this test will become your fitness benchmark. After you progress on to circuit training for your specific chosen sport, every 6-8 weeks you should come back to tackle the Beast again.

By coming this far you have already achieved the hardest task, turned a couch potato into a fit man. It is easy to slip back into indolent ways but sometimes if you have been fit and let it go it's harder to claw that level back again without a specific goal. It's much easier to maintain a consistent routine, exercise three times a week and, if you find yourself slipping, make a real effort to improve your performance.

Remember how difficult it was to begin with? Do you really want to go back to that?

When you get back from your jog or cycle rides write down your intended odd and even exercises on two cards. Put them in transparent plastic bags to keep them waterproof – just in case.

Day 3: The Beast

Go back to your chosen killing field. Don't forget your exercise cards. (If it is really wet underfoot you might want to take a couple of plastic sheets for the floor exercises.) Also remember to take a stop watch.

Warm up for a good 10-15 minutes. Do a few mobilising exercises, jog for 5 minutes, stretch each major muscle group for 10-15 seconds each and then perform each exercise 3 TIMES slowly with a jog between to raise your pulse and body temperature and rehearse the exercises and sequence.

Start at the park bench and **jog** for 10 seconds in a straight line and mark the point exactly, with either a track suit top or the plastic sheet. Leave the even exercise cards (exercises 2,4,6 and so on) at this point and the odd cards (with exercises 1,3,5...) on the park bench as a reminder.

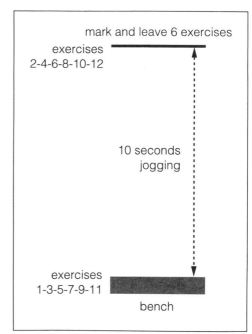

mark and leave 6 exercises
exercises
2-4-6-8-10-12

10 seconds
jogging

exercises
1-3-5-7-9-11

bench

Target Time: 12$\frac{1}{2}$ minutes

Number of circuits: 3 times through

NO STOPPING

Reps per exercise: 12 first circuit
                         10 second circuit
                         12 third circuit

Suggested Circuit

1. Press-ups
2. Half-sits
3. Tuck jumps
4. Clap press-ups
5. Sit-ups with twist
6. Squat thrusts
7. Dips
8. Crunchies
9. Step-ups or Burpees (mandatory in Running Beast)
10. Close arm press-ups
11. Dorsal raises
12. Star jumps

Instructions

Start the watch. Do exercise 1, jog to the marker and do exercise 2 – do it – jog back again to do exercise 3 and so on. Carry on until all 12 exercises have been completed. Then start again doing the number of reps required for each circuit.

Don't be fooled. This is called the Beast because it is a killer. It is relentless. The jogging in between each exercise station gets harder and harder. The intention is to hammer yourself during the exercises and take a rest (!) during the jog. By the third and final circuit – just when you think it's all over and you're going to walk – you will find yourself getting faster again.

The first time out, completing the Beast without stopping during the jog will be an achievement in itself. Make a note of the time you take so you have something to beat on the next outing.

The Running Beast

You might like to test yourself on a rolling interval circuit – our variation on the theme of a running circuit. This is particularly good for training in pairs and small groups for team games. The competitive instinct will drive you on.

Pick a route of a mile round a park or woodland. If you want to be specific about distance, go to a local running track but make sure the grassy areas you choose for the exercises aren't in the middle of the javelin arc! Set your watch to beep at 1-minute intervals.

Jog for 1 minute along the route and when your watch beeps do the exercise. As in the Beast do the same exercises in the same order, except you should replace step-ups with burpees. Change the number of reps to 12, 10, and 8. The incentive is that the faster you do the exercise the longer you get to jog and recover. It's simple but diabolically effective.

Tip

If you want to make the Running Beast more flexible, you can change the time between beeps. Setting it for less than 1 minute makes for a harder workout; setting it for more makes the workout easier.

Motivation Questionnaire

After you have tackled the Beast, ask yourself the following questions:

- Are you able to concentrate for longer periods of time?
- Are you more confident socially, and more relaxed when meeting new people?
- Are you happier and more content?
- Do you feel less tired in the evening after a hard day at work?
- Do you still get headaches after a hard day at work?
- Do you shout at your partner or the kids as much?
- Are you wearing clothes that haven't fitted for a couple of years?
- Do you shake off colds and minor ailments faster?
- Do you still smoke/ have you cut down your drinking?
- Do you think about what you eat?
- Do you enjoy eating your food more and no longer feel guilty about it?
- Has your sex life improved?
- Do people tell you how well or fit you look ?
- Do you like the person you see in the mirror every morning?

There are no right or wrong answers. However, if you have changed at all in the past eight weeks – and you will have done – you should feel a justifiable sense of pride and achievement at what you have achieved.

CONGRATULATIONS!

Maintenance Circuits

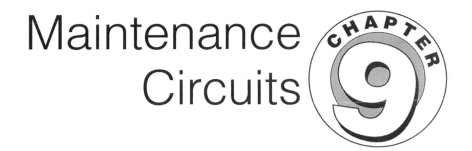

It's all very well getting fit but the hardest part is to maintain your fitness. At this point, the greatest danger is not injury but boredom. Having turned your body from Mr Blobby to Mr Toughy the easiest thing is to rest on your laurels, but if you rest too long on them they will become flabby again. You can certainly take a *few* days off to celebrate, to relax and to let your body rest. A good time unwinding can be worth a week's hard exercise. Remember there is more to life than physical exercise.

You might well consider that you don't want to go all the way. Perhaps you've got to Week 5 on the Nod Circuit Programme and have achieved the level of physical fitness you're happy with. That's fine, different horses... But whatever level you choose to stop at, don't rest for too long – remember that after three weeks off training it takes three days of training to make up for one of laziness. Also don't forget that just because you are exercising less, it doesn't mean you can omit the warm-ups, stretches and cool-downs.

This is just a rule of thumb. The important thing is to feel comfortable – and happy – with your own training schedule. You may not want to train for any particular sport and just wish to keep in shape. But you have to keep interested, doing mental press-ups as well as physical ones. With this in mind, we have devised different approaches to doing circuits, some with different layouts, exercise formats, and variations on a theme. The aim is still to maintain and improve your physical fitness.

The following circuits are suggestions that you can adapt to your own purposes. Refer to the index of circuit exercises at the back of the book (which are graded – Easy, Tough, and Killer) if you want to choose different exercises. The only rule to follow is stick to the ATL (Arm, Trunk, Leg) approach and always include one lower back (dorsal) exercise per circuit.

Suggested circuit (Hard)

1 Dips
2 Sit-ups with twist
3 Alternate squat thrusts
4 Clap press-ups
5 Dorsal presses
6 Star jumps
7 Wide arm press-ups
8 V-sits
9 Squats or step-ups
10 Close arm press-ups
11 Crunchies
12 Dorsal raises

Cone Sprint Circuit

Choose your exercises using the ATL approach. You need 6 for the first circuit, 9 for the second and 12 for the third. Either remember (!) or write down the exercises on a piece of paper or card or a chalkboard. You also need a 20-metre stretch of grass, track or concrete. Place a mat (blanket or equivalent) at the start, then the first cone (shirt or other object to hand) at 10 metres, a second at 15 metres and a third at 20 metres. Place a bench behind the mat for step-ups and dips.

Instructions

First circuit: 10 reps per exercise
Second circuit: 8 reps per exercise
Third circuit: 6 reps per exercise

NO REST BETWEEN EXERCISES
NO REST BETWEEN CIRCUITS

Do all the exercises on the mat. After each exercise sprint to the nearest cone, run around it and sprint back to the mat for the next exercise. On the second circuit, run around the second cone (15 metres away). On the third circuit, run around the third cone. If this proves too much, you might want to reverse the order, decreasing the sprint distances as you get tired. In other words, run around the third cone on the first circuit.

Variation Do the circuit with a partner. While one of you sprints, the other performs the exercise. Change when your partner reaches the mat after running around the cone. The faster the partner sprints, the fewer exercises you have to perform. If you want your partner to work harder, just jog around the cone – although you must be prepared to pay for the consequences.

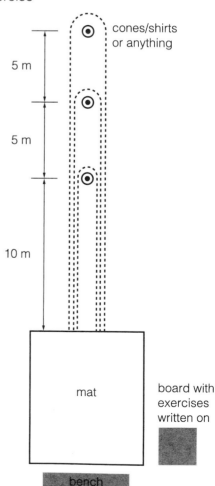

Cross-Country Circuit

This is very tough so it is only suitable for those of higher fitness levels. But it is great fun. Variety will enhance this circuit whereas a lack of imagination will stifle it. If you go out expecting to get down and dirty, puffed and soggy you will find this enjoyable, flexible, interesting and very tough.

Instructions

Choose 9 or 12 exercises according to the ATL approach.
Allow 15-20 seconds per exercise.
NO REST BETWEEN EXERCISES
You may rest between circuits for 60 seconds if you wish.

Find a small cross-country route a minimum of 200 metres. It needs to have something to jump over (a bench or a nice deep puddle), something to go under, a nice boggy bit, plus trees to weave in and out of. In fact anything that needs to be tackled, makes you work and gets you nice and muddy (so don't wear brand new kit).

The course could require such extras as:

- Vaulting over gates.
- Crawling under gates.
- Weaving in and out of trees.
- Running along park benches (make sure they are not occupied).
- Scaling walls.
- Balancing along the top of walls.
- Being chased by a dog (!).
- Jumping puddles.

After the first circuit of 9 or 12 exercises run around the route.
After the second circuit run around the route going the other way.
After the third circuit run around the route both ways. If you think it will help, make a note of your total time and aim to beat it next time.

Variation: Do an exercise after each obstacle – for instance run along a wall, hit the ground and do your press-ups.

It is difficult to recommend a specific exercise circuit as this will depend on what apparatus you find along your route and your fitness level. However, it could include such exercises as:
- Dips on bench.
- Pull-ups on branches – be careful they don't break.
- Sergeant jumps against walls.
- Press-ups in water.
- Raised leg press-ups using gate bar.
- Squat thrusts over a puddle.
- Running up streams.

Star Circuit

This is a circuit that is best suited to a gym and a larger group of people. Choose any 10 exercises (following the ATL approach) and arrange 10 exercise stations. They should all be 5 metres from a centre point.

Instructions

Start at Station 1 and do 15 seconds of reps of the specified exercise. At the whistle blast (or beep of your watch if you are doing it solo), sprint to the centre point, touch it and sprint back to Station 2. And so on. Do the circuit 3 times. Breaks between circuits can be up to a minute depending on fitness level.

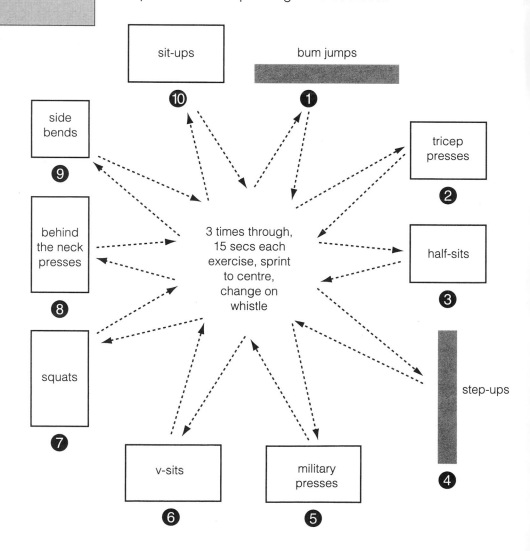

Sprint Killer Circuit

This circuit is also suited to a larger group of individuals as it takes some effort to set it out. Ideally it should be done in a gym but if you are outside you need a 20-50 x 10 metre stretch of flat ground.

Measure out 9 exercise stations of your choice (using the ATL approach) at roughly equal intervals between the start and the chosen finish. Place a row of benches or a piece of string as a marker 5 metres away from the stations.

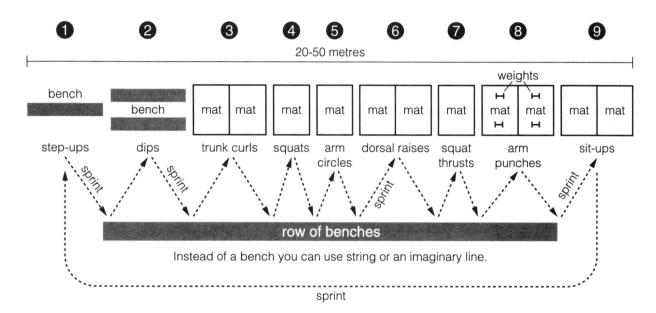

Instructions

Spend 10 seconds at each station. Sprint to the bench or line marker. When you have done the exercises at Station 9, sprint to the start. 30 seconds rest between circuits. Do 3 circuits.

Suggested Circuit (Easy)

1 Step-ups
2 Dips
3 Trunk curls
4 Squats
5 Arm circles
6 Dorsal raises
7 Squat thrusts
8 Arm punches
9 Sit-ups

Overload Circuit

This is a change from the normal routine in that you beast each part of your body and then move on to the next.

Choose 9 exercises: 3 arm (including 1 dorsal exercise), 3 trunk and 3 leg. Place 3 exercise stations each 10 metres apart.

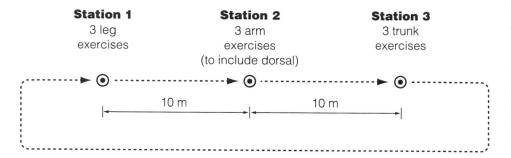

Station 1
3 leg
exercises

Station 2
3 arm
exercises
(to include dorsal)

Station 3
3 trunk
exercises

10 m   10 m

Instructions

Complete 3 leg exercises at Station 1.
Sprint to Station 2.
Complete 3 arm exercises.
Sprint to Station 3.
Complete 3 trunk exercises.
Sprint back to Station 1.

Allow 15 seconds for each exercise.
Alternatively, allow 20 seconds for the first
    circuit, 15 seconds for the second, and
    10 for the third.
NO REST BETWEEN CIRCUITS
Do 3 times through.

Suggested Circuit (Intermediate)

Station 1
Tuck jumps
Squat thrusts
Burpees

Station 2
Press-ups
Dorsal raises
Arm punches

Station 3
V-sits
Half-sits
Crunchies

Sports Specific Circuits

Now you're fit and you've beaten the Beast. But one reason you might have taken up this serious exercise in the first place was that you were tired with being thrashed by that so-called friend at tennis or squash, or you're fed up with flailing around as your Sunday soccer team gets stuffed by the local pub team. You know you can beat them; it's always close but somehow in those dying minutes you've never had the strength. Well now you have, and it's time to use your fitness to improve your individual sports skills.

We have selected and designed circuits for some of the most popular sporting activities in Britain. Not everybody plays rugby or cricket so we also show how you can work out your own circuit to fit the specifications of the sport you want to pursue.

Many of these circuits are based on those designed by Marine PTIs to train large groups of men so they can be carried out by entire teams. If you want to train for rugby on your own, you may have to adapt the demands of the circuit to suit your requirements. Some of the circuits require specific equipment but this shouldn't be difficult to obtain.

Whatever sport you play, we suggest that you read the first four circuits (rugby, football, skiing and racquet sports). They explain how each exercise can help to improve your performance in the specific sport.

Rugby Circuit

Rugby fitness is not only multi-dimensional, it also varies according to the player's position on the field and the fitness demands of the game. Fitness tests can be used to assess a player's strengths and weaknesses in order to structure a programme that is relevant to the individual. As with most sports there is no better way to develop fitness than specific circuit training and resistance work.

This is a circuit of various techniques and exercise theories that Dieter has found to be a great success. It is designed to be used by first and second teams and can have as many as 30 players exercising at once – if you double up the exercise stations. All the running exercises can be performed with or without a ball. The circuit is designed to produce muscular endurance and strength in the entire body.

The time spent on each exercise depends on the fitness of the players. Start with 15-20 seconds at each station for the first time through, and 30 seconds on each station for the next circuit. They should run back to the start in 15-20 seconds so they can blast it out for the final circuit. If everyone is up to it, there is no harm in doing a fourth circuit.

Instructions

Warm-up: 10 minutes
Circuit: 17-18 minutes
Changes on a whistle blast

Station 1: Alternate shoulder presses

The nature of the game lends itself to a lot of running hand-offs and shoulder tackles. Shoulder presses develop upper-body power and muscular endurance if you use small weights and lots of reps. (To develop strength use heavier weights and fewer reps.)

Station 2: Crunchies

These develop strong abdominal muscles, which work whenever the trunk is being used. The exercise should be done slowly to improve strength, and quickly to improve endurance. Breathe out every time you come up. Being tackled takes a lot out of the body – especially head on. Good abs mean you can take harder knocks on tackles from the front.

Station 3: Squats with bar

These should be performed slowly and will develop power and strength in the legs and lower back. Any pack member will agree the stronger the legs, the longer the drive.

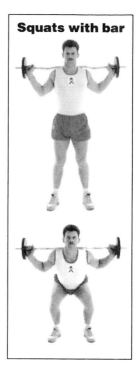

Squats with bar

Station 4: Press-ups

These are great for all players because they develop muscular endurance of the arms and chest. They will also improve upper-body strength.

Station 5: Alternate V-sits

Lift one leg and both arms to touch the shin, lower under control and change legs. Ensure you breathe out on the way up and in on the way down. This exercise develops strength in the abs and hip flexors which are most important when sprinting or driving forward. It can be performed while holding a ball in your hands.

Station 6: Burpees

Go down to a crouch, push the legs out to the press-ups position. Go back to the crouch then stand up. Burpees provide a good all-over body workout that can be completed without any equipment. They help to improve coordination as well as fitness.

Station 7: Lateral raises

Raise arms with weights to just over shoulder height and lower under control. This will develop the lateral part of the shoulders, which helps improve strength and muscular endurance.

Station 8: Half-sits

These should be done slowly to improve strength in your abs and quickly to improve endurance.

Station 9: Squat thrusts

This is a good general body exercise that can be performed without equipment. Your knees can come inside or outside your arms. Squat thrusts work the shoulders in a static position and work the hip flexors and quads in an explosive action, promoting muscular endurance in the hips.

Station 10: Dips

Like alternate shoulder presses, these will develop power and muscular endurance in the arms.

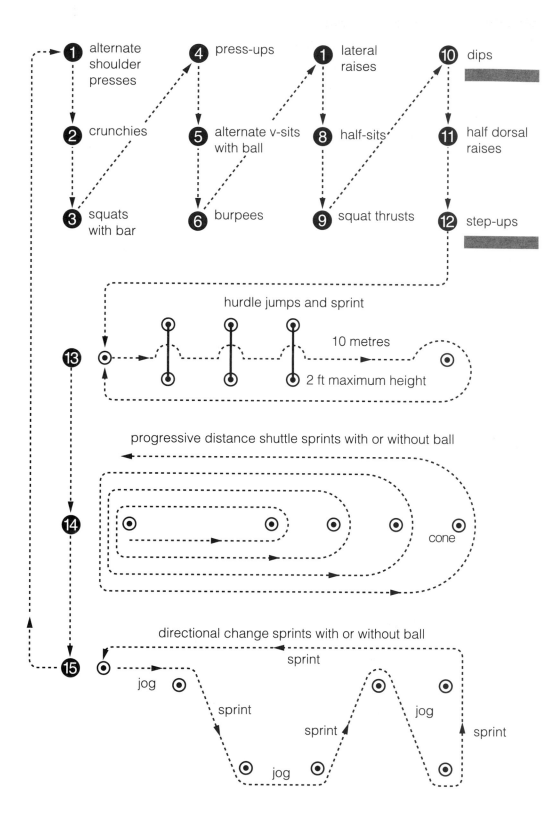

alternate shoulder presses — 1

press-ups — 4

lateral raises — 1

dips — 10

crunchies — 2

alternate v-sits with ball — 5

half-sits — 8

half dorsal raises — 11

squats with bar — 3

burpees — 6

squat thrusts — 9

step-ups — 12

hurdle jumps and sprint

10 metres

2 ft maximum height

13

progressive distance shuttle sprints with or without ball

14

cone

directional change sprints with or without ball

15

sprint

jog

sprint

sprint

jog

jog

sprint

Station 11: Half dorsal raises

Many players work their abs without balancing them out with exercises for the lower back. This exercise supports the whole back with the majority of work done on the lower back.

Station 12: Step-ups

The box or bench should not be over 35 cm (14 inches) high and you should put your whole foot on it. This exercise works the major leg muscles and the hip flexors, both of which are used when sprinting or driving forward.

The Power and Endurance Phase

The last three exercises develop a player's aerobic and anaerobic capabilities. Rugby is not played at one steady speed but involves both short power sprints of various distances and directional change.

Station 13: Hurdle jumps and sprint

Place hurdles, no more than 60 cm (2 ft) high, 1 metre apart. Have your feet comfortably apart. Jump over first hurdle, on landing jump up and over the next hurdle and so on. Drive knees up and swing arms forwards. On the last jump, sprint to the cone (10 metres away). Jog back to the start and repeat. This exercise develops pure power and strength in the quadriceps. It also helps you speed around the pitch.

Station 14: Progressive shuttle sprints (with or without ball)

Place four cones 10 metres apart. Sprint up to the first cone, then jog back to the start, turn and sprint back to the second cone and so on. When you reach the final cone, jog back to the start and repeat. Here, you will be using all your lower limb muscles. This session produces leg power at varying distances but at the same speed, which is good for both forwards and backs.

Station 15: Directional change sprint (with or without ball)

Rugby is not a one-directional game. You have to be able to change direction and speed instantly. Place six cones in whatever position you require. Jog to the first cone, sprint to the second, jog to the third, sprint to the fourth and so on. At the sixth cone, sprint to the finish and repeat the sequence again. This helps to build up sprinting power and the muscles that initiate directional change. Again, you will be using all the lower limb muscles.

Football Circuit

Although it is a team game, football requires a very special mix of aerobic and anaerobic fitness depending on the needs of each player. The circuit is controlled by a whistle blast to change each exercise. Each station can take up to two players so 22 players can train together. Each exercise can last as long as you want but start with 15-25 seconds per station for the first run through, 30-40 for the second and 15-20 for the third.

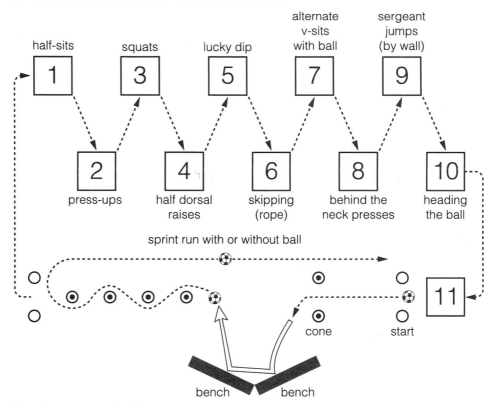

Station 1: Half-sits
These develop muscular endurance in the abdominals. They are useful exercises because the abs play a big part in posture and in movements on the field.

Station 2: Press-ups
Press-ups improve upper-body strength and, while they are essential for all sports, power in the triceps can be a benefit for throw-ins and goalkeepers.

Station 3: Squats
Perform these slowly and use weights if you wish. Footballers are known for having strong quads. Squats strengthen these muscles and will increase running power.

Station 4: Half dorsal raises

Strong dorsals will support the back on throws when the player pushes his hips forwards and the ball is passed over his head. Generally, you should do one dorsal exercise for every three abdominal exercises.

Station 5: Lucky dip

Choose 4 trunk/arm exercises and write each on a piece of card. Lay these face down on the floor/ground. Each player picks one and does that exercise. This gives variety and improves upper body strength and endurance.

Station 6: Skipping

Skipping with a rope develops cardiovascular fitness and good body coordination. Both factors are needed on the pitch.

Station 7: Alternate v-sits (with ball)

Lie down with arms and legs extended, holding the ball in both hands. Lift one leg and both arms with the ball, touch the ball at the laces or shin, bending in the middle. This develops coordination, and strength in the abs and hip flexors which are important when sprinting.

Station 8: Behind the neck presses

These improve upper-body strength. Power in the triceps can be a benefit for throw-ins and goalkeepers.

Station 9: Sergeant jumps

These help to improve power in the quadriceps in ballistic movements as in heading the ball and kicking.

Station 10: Heading the ball

This is to improve coordination and ball control on eye-to-ball contact. Head the ball against a wall or between partners. Or throw the ball for your partner to aim at a goal and then swap roles.

Station 11: Sprint run (with or without ball)

The player either runs from the start with a ball to the first set of cones, passes the ball to the benches and back to himself, then dribbles through the cones, sprints back to the start and repeats. If without a ball, he jogs to first cones, sprints to the zig-zag of cones, then back to the start and repeats. This exercise works both the aerobic and anaerobic systems of the player in a way similar to the flow of the game.

Skiing Circuit

Having spent years perfecting his own technique on the slopes and recovering from soreness and bruising, Corporal 'Jumper' Collin developed ski fitness classes. He was then approached by the Royal Navy/Marines ski team to help them in 1993-94 when they achieved good championship results. This circuit can be done either by a team or a lone worker. The exercises are devised as a total body conditioner and leg workout.

Instructions

To get maximum benefit from the circuit, do 15-20 reps on the legs, 20-25 on the trunk and 10-15 on arm exercises. Perform each exercise then sprint to the centre cone and back to the next station.

Complete 3-4 whole circuits with a rest of 1 minute between each one. If using this as a group circuit, let everyone exercise for about 20-30 seconds at each station and move on to the next on a whistle blast. If people are doubled up the circuit can take a maximum load of 18 people.

Station 1: Arm swings

When doing these, lean forwards to emulate a ski position. Bend your arms and *control* the swing of the weights forwards and backwards to simulate the skiing action. Once you are in a rhythm the exercise is easier.

Station 2: Half v-sits

These are a good way to strengthen and firm up the trunk – essential for skiing where the whole body needs to be conditioned.

Station 3: Squats

In skiing you very rarely stand completely upright, generally you are in a semi-squat. Try to emulate this position to develop good leg strength and power through the same range of movement you use on the slopes. Your legs should be just over a shoulder-width apart. Keep the back straight as you go down into the squat. From there straighten the knees slightly into a semi-squat position. Perform the action slowly.

Station 4: Arm punches

Do these while leaning forwards in a ski position. This exercise builds up strength in the upper body, which will benefit most skiers whether it be lifting themselves out of a snowdrift or pole planting.

Station 5: Half dorsal raises

Because of the skier's basic position, the lower back takes a lot of punishment. These will strengthen it and delay the onset of pain during a hard ski.

Station 6: Floor touches

Direction change at speed is hard to emulate during an exercise. Mark a line on the floor and stand with your legs apart, feet either side of it. Place two cones about 60-90 cm (2-3 ft) out of arm's reach at either side. Lean over to one side and touch the cone – then back to the other side. Try not to cross the line. Remain side on to the cone.

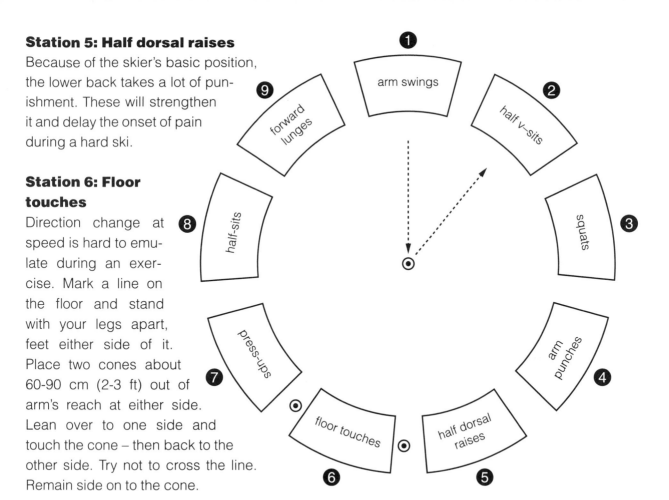

Station 7: Press-ups

Press-ups improve upper-body strength and endurance – useful when pole planting and cross-country skiing.

Station 8: Half-sits

Good abdominal control is needed in skiing. Strong abs help hold the position on the downhill dash for longer without extra strain on the lower back.

Station 9: Forward lunges

These are essential for Telemark skiers and downhillers. They develop strength and power in the quadriceps.

Racquet Sports Circuit

This circuit is relevant to all racquet sports – squash, tennis, table tennis, badminton, rackets, and real tennis. It is designed to be a fun circuit that combines skill, strength and agility – three vital components that you need for all racquet, eye-to-ball contact games. The fun aspect should not deter the player to work less hard, because the harder he works, the more fatigued he becomes and so his coordination and reactions become slower.

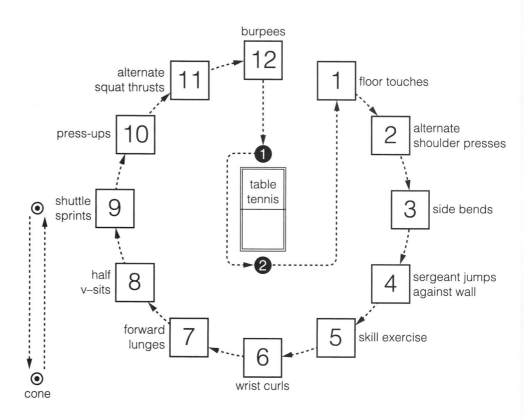

Instructions

20 seconds per exercise
10 seconds rest between each exercise
3 circuits
30 seconds rest between circuits

There should be one person at each exercise station and two at the table in the centre. Everyone exercises and the two in the centre play for the length of time determined for the whistle change. Then everyone moves around one station. Player 1 goes round the table to take player 2's place and so on. (The table tennis table could be swapped for a badminton net.) If you cannot rustle up 14 people it is possible to do it with as few as two with a little bit of working out. By yourself you might wish to adapt it to a squash circuit: try hitting a ball against a wall in place of the table tennis.

Station 1: Floor touches

This exercise is to develop muscular reaction and stability at speed. Mark a line on the floor and stand with your legs apart feet either side of the line. Place two cones about 60-90 cm (2-3 ft) out of arm's reach at either side. The object is to not cross the line and to remain side on to the cone. Lean down and touch the cone – then back to the other side. Try not to cross the line at any time. You can perform the exercise with a racquet in the hand – every time you come to the upright position change arms with the racquet.

Station 2: Alternate shoulder presses

These strengthen the shoulder muscles and shoulder girdle, which particularly benefits the player during the serve and volley actions – where the muscle is put under great strain.

Station 3: Side bends

This exercise works the oblique muscles, which play a major part in the actions of serving, lunging with your racquet extended, and turning to hit a ball or shuttlecock. Players often overlook this simple exercise and in doing so they risk injury and having to take time off from the game. Lean directly over to each side in turn and try to touch your knee or further down.

Station 4: Sergeant jumps

These develop strength, power and test the muscles to fatigue level. Movement across the court can be multi-directional and at varying speeds. The power in the legs in explosive take-offs emulates this rapid change in movement. Sergeant jumps have to be performed near a wall. You need a mark on the floor and another on the wall. Jump up to touch the mark on the wall (usually 2.4-2.7 metres/8-9 ft high) then down to the floor (60-90 cm/2-3 ft from the start mark).

Station 5: Skill exercise

This exercise develops eye-to-ball coordination and strengthens the forearm muscles. By now you should be tired and your concentration flagging. Take a table-tennis bat or the racquet of your choice. Aim to keep a ball or shuttlecock in the air by turning the racquet forward and back, striking the object backhand and forehand – as if you were flipping a pancake in a frying pan.

To make the exercise more difficult, mark out a route (using cones etc) and walk or jog round it as you flip your bat or racquet.

Station 6: Wrist curls
All racquet sports demand great power in the wrist and forearm to be able to strike the ball with power and accuracy without losing the grip. Keep the elbow as still as possible as you flex the wrist.

Station 7: Forward lunges
These develop muscle power when the body is in full stretch. Strength is required to stand with back upright and repeat the action in another direction. Keep body upright as you lunge forwards.

Station 8: Half v-sits
The whole body needs to be conditioned for all sports. This is one of the best ways of strengthening and firming up the trunk. Try to work all the body parts as this will improve your game.

Station 9: Shuttle sprints
Place two cones 20-30 metres apart. Sprint to each cone, touch it and sprint back. Carry a racquet as you run.

In squash especially the cardiovascular system is worked to the maximum. Short rallies and sprints are in the nature of the game, so it is imperative to develop cardiovascular fitness. Remember the old adage 'get fit to play squash, don't play squash to get fit'.

Station 10: Press-ups
Upper-body strength is essential with most racquet sports. If you condition your body so you can sustain play over long periods and resist the various pressures put on it, you will be able to outlast and beat a more naturally skilful opponent.

Station 11: Alternate squat thrusts
These develop coordination between the leg movements at speed – something people take for granted until they try. They help to develop strength and power in the hip flexors.

Station 12: Burpees
Burpees improve cardiovascular endurance, develop muscular endurance in the lower limbs and promote coordination. Go down to a crouch, push the legs out to the press-ups position, back to the crouch, then stand up. Repeat in a fluid motion.

Running Circuit

This is simple circuit designed to improve your muscular endurance for running. It makes a change to vary your training regime – you could do this to prevent boredom on a long run and to reduce the time you spend in the gym.

Instructions
20 seconds per exercise
3 times through
1 minute between circuits

After each circuit finish with 40 seconds each of these exaggerated movements:

Bounding: Keep off the ground as much as possible, like the
    step in a triple jump.
High leg raises: Run with knees coming up towards the chin.
High hell kicking: Run with heels coming up to the backside.
Skipping: Like a kid.

1 10-metre **shuttle sprint**
2 **Sit-ups with twist**
3 **Shoulder shrugs** (with weights)
4 **Tuck jumps**
5 **Dorsal raises**
6 **Dips**
7 **Alternate squat thrusts**
8 **Crunchies**
9 **Arm running action** (with weights)

Basketball Circuit

This is a simple circuit for anyone who wants to get fitter for basketball. If possible use a court or an area with similar dimensions. Take a basketball with you.

Instructions
20 seconds per exercise
3 times through
1 minute between circuits

1 **Shuttle sprint** over 10 metres (dribbling or running with ball as option)
2 **Alternate dorsal raises**
3 **Close arm press-ups** (hands on basketball as option)
4 **Sergeant jumps**
5 **Sit-ups with twist** (use ball to touch floor on either side of leg, if you wish)
6 **Military presses** with barbell or ball to chest (very fast)
7 **Bastards**
8 **V-sits** (using ball to touch toes, if you wish)
9 **Clap press-ups**

Finish with full court dribbling and shooting 10 times.

SPORTS SPECIFIC CIRCUITS

Golf Circuit

Although golf as a recreational activity is rarely associated with fitness training, competitive golf requires a high standard of fitness, and particularly local muscle endurance. If you want to increase cardiovascular intensity, space exercise stations 20 metres apart and jog in between. Even tougher, after each exercise carry a full golf bag and jog between stations!

Instructions

20 seconds per exercise

3 times through

1 minute between circuits

Finish each circuit with 25 swings of a wood. Then start again.

1 **Weight winding on rope**
2 **Sit-ups with twist**
3 **Step-ups**
4 **Lateral raises**
5 **Dorsal raises**
6 **Squats**
7 **Arm curls**
8 **Standing twists** (holding golf club behind neck if you wish)
9 **Dips**

Swimming Circuit

Swimming is superb exercise in that it demands all-round fitness. This is a swimming circuit you can do out of the water! To increase the intensity of the circuit, try swimming across the pool after each exercise. The Royal Marines swimming teams do this at least once a week – and it's a real killer.

Instructions

3 times through

10 seconds per exercise for sprint swimmers

15-20 seconds per exercise for endurance swimmers

Between circuits: 30 seconds rest for sprint swimmers

No rest for endurance swimmers

1 **Close arm press-ups**
2 **Dorsal raises**
3 **Alternate squat thrusts**
4 **Raised leg press-ups**
5 **Crunchies with twist**
6 **Toe tapping** on raised bench/platform 30 cm (12 inches) high
7 **Dips**
8 **Side bends**
9 **Flutter/scissor kicks**
10 **Arm swimming action** (your choice) using light weights
11 **V-sits**
12 **Tuck jumps**

Multi-Gym Circuit

This circuit is ideal for people who spend a lot of time travelling on business and end up staying in hotels. Many hotels have an exercise room but machines vary and they can be a daunting sight to the uninitiated.

Before embarking on this circuit recce the machines (they often have a diagram stuck on the wall which may or may not be comprehensible). Try them out to get to know the action needed to perform an exercise. Always follow the safety guidelines and, if in doubt, seek the advice of a qualified instructor. The circuit is designed for a simple all-round workout. As you get to know the machines and muscle groups involved you can invent your own circuit using the ATL approach.

Make sure you go through a warm-up and stretch routine. If you have come off a long plane journey take extra care to make sure you are hydrated, and warm up and stretch for longer than normal.

Use very light weights – you must be able to perform all 12 exercises without too much gritting of teeth, holding breath, screaming or cheating!

Instructions

12 exercises
20 seconds per exercise
3 times through
No rest between exercises
No rest between circuits
(depending on fitness –
take 1 minute if you
feel you need it)

Shoulder presses
Main muscles used: deltoids; trapezius; triceps

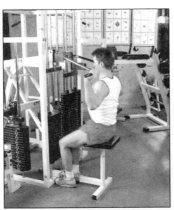
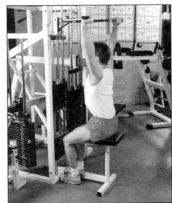

Incline sit-ups
Main muscles used: abdominals; hip flexors

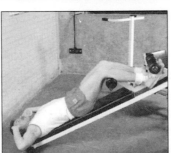
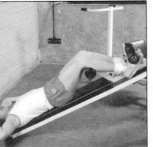
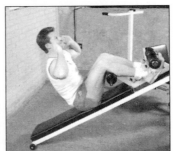

Leg presses

Main muscles used: quadriceps; calf muscles

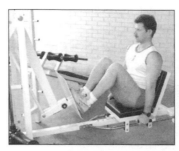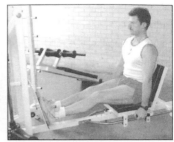

Upright rowing

Main muscles used: trapezius; deltoids

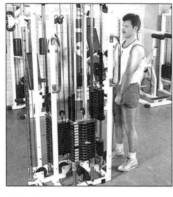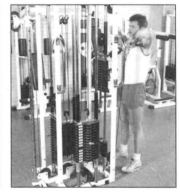

Now do **sit-ups** on a flat bench or floor mat
Main muscles used: abdominals; hip flexors

Hamstring curls

Main muscles used: hamstrings; gluteals

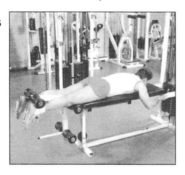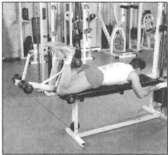

Now do **dorsal raises** on a flat bench or floor mat
Main muscles used: lower back; deltoids

Lat pull-downs

Main muscles used: upper back

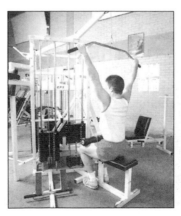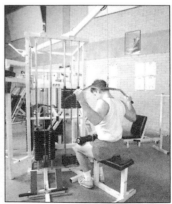

Leg extensions
Main muscles used: quadriceps

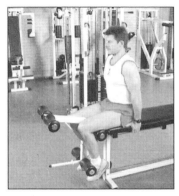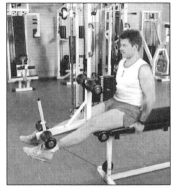

Bench presses
Main muscles used: pectorals; biceps

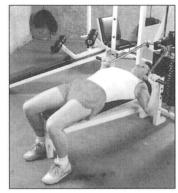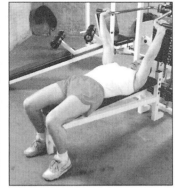

Hip flexion
Main muscles used: hip flexors; abdominals (statically)

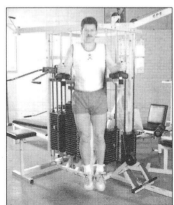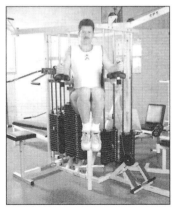

Calf raises
Main muscles used: calf muscles

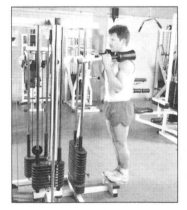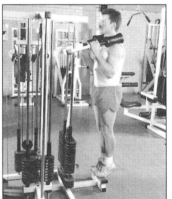

Cricket Circuit

Cricket is a skills-oriented game requiring both mental and physical fitness. This circuit alternates skills with free-standing exercises thrown in to improve general fitness levels. It requires a minimum of two players but can incorporate a full team. You will need basic cricket equipment plus a few extras.

Instructions

Do circuit twice (note that different stations require different times)
No rest between exercises (go straight on to next one and put on kit asap)
2 minutes rest between circuits

Station 1: Dips

10-20 reps, depending on fitness level.

Station 2: Batting skills (2 players): 2 minutes

After striking the ball, the batsman runs 5 metres to a line and returns. He must play the ball either back to bowler or to another target (like an old box) to encourage accurate batting. The bowler can try to get the batsman out.

Station 3: Half-sits with twist

Holding bat! 15-25 reps.

Station 4: Pick up and run: 2 minutes

Place balls between two lines 20 metres apart. Pick up ball and run to the other line. Place ball down and repeat using different hand for pick up. Partner can either replace balls or run in opposite direction!

Station 5: Arm punches

Using bat held in both hands, punch arms for 30-45 seconds.

Station 6: Bean bag bowl (2 players): 2 minutes

To improve bowling skills, bowl bean bags at a target. No rest for 2 minutes, using full run up and correct bowling action. Partner feeds/replaces bags.

Station 7: Squat thrusts

30-45 seconds, depending on fitness level.

Station 8: Catching skills: 2 minutes

Throw a tennis ball against a wall, getting further away and then coming back in. You can also do this with partner or a slip catch machine if you have one.

Station 9: Standing twists holding bat behind neck

30-45 seconds.

Station 10: Running skills (2 players): 30 seconds

Place two lines wicket-distance apart. Race partner for 30 seconds carrying bat (pads optional). Ground bat as you would to score a run. The object is to score more runs than your partner.

Station 11: Air strokes

30-45 seconds of air strokes with bat, or hit soft tennis balls bowled by a partner. Choose your own strokes but change every five shots.

Station 12: Fielding skills (2 players): 2 minutes

Standing by the wicket or target, one player (wicket-keeping gloves or baseball mitt optional) should roll the ball in any direction towards a line 20-25 metres away. The partner tries to stop the ball reaching the line, pick up – and, if required, throw the ball at the target.

Cycling Circuit

This circuit is designed to improve the performance of cyclists at three levels. It's something to do when it's snowing or raining too hard for all but the two-wheeled fanatic. A good alternative circuit, it can also be done in a gym (don't forget to cycle there and back)! Include exercises on a stationary bike if possible as part of your warm-up and cool-down.

Instructions

Do circuit three times
15 seconds each exercise (fanatics do 30 seconds for all *leg* exercises)
No rest between exercises

Exercises 1-6: Pleasure cyclists (1 minute between circuits)
Exercises 1-9: Fitness through cycling (30 seconds between circuits)
Exercises 1-12: Competitive cyclists (no rest between circuits)

1 **Wide arm press-ups**
2 **Sit-ups with twist**
3 **Alternate squat thrusts**
4 **Dips**
5 **Crunchies**
6 **Tuck jumps or burpees**
7 **Pull-ups/ Lat pull-downs**
    (multi-gym exercise)
8 **Dorsal presses**
9 **Calf raises**
10 **Raised leg press-ups**
11 **Half-sits**
12 **Star jumps**

Boxing Circuit

Boxing is a very individual sport and still incredibly popular despite all the adverse press and media speculation following various tragedies in the ring. Boxercise classes are enjoyed by both men and women, mainly because of the variety of basic exercises that make the participants work to their maximum. The beauty of this workout is that it is both fun and physically demanding. You have a hard workout followed by periods of rest, which can be varied according to individual fitness and ability. If possible you should aim to get some basic specialist boxing training to enhance your performance and reduce the risk of injury. This is best carried out in a gym unless you have a punching bag and machines at home.

Instructions

The circuit follows the format of a boxing match with 3 minutes of work in each round. Depending on your fitness level you can go through as many rounds as you want. 10 rounds will come to 30 minutes work, 10 minutes rest – a 40-minute workout that will prove very rewarding… and tiring.

Round 1 is three exercises which you rotate after 1 minute

No rest between exercises

1 minute rest between rounds

Round 1

Skipping: Try to maintain a steady rhythm. This not only develops physical fitness but aids total coordination. The heart and lungs work intensely over the minute, the shoulders work to maintain the skipping action.

Crunchies: This is a good exercise for a boxer who has to protect himself from blows to the abdomen. An increase in muscle strength can help this area and make the boxer into a more formidable opponent.

Behind the neck presses: Ensure you have a weight you can control for a minute's work. When wearing 14-16 oz gloves and blocking and throwing punches, the arms feel heavy within seconds. You require good endurance work over the shoulder girdle.

Round 2

Step-ups: Using a box or aerobics step (maximum height 35 cm/14 inches), step on and off ensuring heels are on the box. Do fast or slow. Overall fitness is required for sport, and strong legs that don't fatigue quickly play an important part.

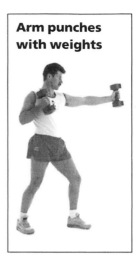

Arm punches with weights

Incline press-ups: Place hands on bench or step-up box, lower until chest is just over box then raise to full extension. Press-ups are a great muscular endurance exercise for the upper body. By raising the body and putting the hands on the box, the exercise becomes easier so you can perform quality press-ups for the full minute.

Punch bag: Stand arm's reach from bag, leading foot forward. Jab the bag with the leading hand then the other. Depending on skill you can add a combination of punches. This is where specialist training comes in – the better you are, the harder you work. If you want to relieve stress there is no better exercise. Remember bag mitts are essential to reduce injury.

Round 3

Half-sits: Lie down, hands on thighs, lift head and shoulders, slide hands up to knees, and breathe out. Lower and repeat for 1 minute. These strengthen the abdominals (see Crunchies in Round 1).

Skipping: Try to maintain a steady rhythm (see Round 1).

Arm punches: Stand in boxing stance with a light weight in both hands. Punch continuously to the front, changing stance and style if you wish. This develops the serratus anterior – the punching muscle. There is no better way to strengthen any muscle than to take it through its action and full range of movement under an exercise with stress (in this case weights).

Variation: This is an alternative boxing circuit with just four exercises repeated and no rest between except if you finish the shoulder presses, upright rowing and Nieder press in under 1 minute. This is very demanding. Try it – it's awesome!

Instructions
Do six times – no stopping
Station 1: Skipping 1 minute
Station 2: Crunchies 1 minute
Station 3: Alternate shoulder presses x 10 reps
    Upright rowing x 10 reps,
    Nieder presses x 10. Complete in under 1 minute, remaining time is rest!
Station 4: Punch bag 1 minute

How to design your own circuit

Not everyone plays cricket, soccer or tennis. Although we have included lots of circuits in this book, you might want to create your own version, geared towards your favourite sport. The way to do this is to analyse your own particular activity and from that you can devise your own circuit programme. First ask yourself the following questions:

1 What major and minor muscle groups are used?

The muscle groups used will determine the main exercises to be performed – this acts as a good starting point – but after you have answered the next questions, the number of exercises will probably have to be whittled down. Concentrate on the main muscle groups before looking at the minor ones.

2 What action is used? How is the muscle used?

What is it? Kicking, jumping, throwing, cycling? What is the arm action? This will also help in determining the type of exercise.

3 What component of physical fitness is needed? Strength, endurance, power, speed, motor fitness or a combination?

Deciding on the component of physical fitness will determine the format of the circuit. Is flexibility a real issue? If so, put in more stretching.

In squash, motor fitness is important so can you replicate that in a circuit? Yes – by using the racquet and ball between exercises. Keep the ball up at the end of the circuit and hit it against a wall 10 times. Practise strokes with a partner and get him to play certain shots for you to return.

Is strength an issue? If so, use weights.

Is endurance an issue? If so, increase the number of reps.

4 How long is the activity/sport?

The duration of the event will determine how long you want to work out for.

For football, obviously you don't want to work out for 90 minutes but you may want the whole process to last a little longer than normal. So throw in a short kick-about as a warm-up, thereby adding to the time. Generally in football you will work hard in short bursts for 10-20 seconds then rest. Therefore keep your reps time down to this length of time.

5 How important is skill in the activity?

If skill is very important you may wish to put more skills-related activities into the circuit, interspersing with basic circuit exercises (eg cricket circuit).

6 Are there any rests during the activity? If so, how long do you have to get your breath back (eg between rallies, between a play in rugby/football)?

Rests in the activity will help to determine rest time in the circuit, both in between exercises and circuits. Tennis is a sport where there are short bursts of intense activity – turning, running, ground and overhead strokes – followed by a rest between points. So consider having longer exercise periods of 20-30 seconds, followed by pauses between exercises.

7 What are your favourite exercises?

Everyone has their favourite exercises. There is no harm in using personal preferences but keep a balance. Spread the muscle group overload.

Once you have taken all these questions into consideration, you can devise a well-balanced workout to suit your exact needs.

Devising your circuit

This is the hard part. Try to stick to 9 exercises at first, following the ATL rotation. This will give you enough of a variety to prevent the circuit from becoming monotonous. Remember that the exercises have to be related to the sport. For example, hockey requires leg and arm strength, endurance and coordination. When you feel happy with 9 exercises, consider increasing it to 12.

Layout

The circuit layout should be easy to follow. Keep it in a logical sequence eg **1** Press-ups (Arms); **2** Sit-ups (Trunk); **3** Squats (Legs) and so on. This ensures a good all-round body workout. Keep it simple – the simplest circuits are often the hardest. Concentrate on doing the full range of exercises.

Remember the WBA

Treat the body as a whole. Don't just work out and strengthen the parts you think you need to concentrate on. For instance, on first analysis a cyclist might think he should just concentrate on his legs and ignore his lower back. But he also needs a strong lower back as he is bent over the bike putting perpetual strain on that area for hours at a time. Balance is the key.

Timing

The length of circuit depends on your level of fitness. However, remember you need 21 minutes to get real benefit from the exercises. So 3 times through 9 exercises at 30 seconds each is only $13\frac{1}{2}$ minutes work.

Don't Forget

Remember to warm up and cool down and build gradually to a longer circuit. You can always break the circuit exercises with a few minutes of a skill exercise.

The SBS Challenge

CHAPTER 11

Note

While passing this test means you are a very fit bastard it does not mean you would be accepted into the SBS. They are looking for other qualities as well... and the selection procedure gets tougher and tougher.

So, if you've still got the stamina and fitness, it's time for the SBS challenge. This Test is based on the initial physical tests that any Marine who wishes to join the SBS has to pass before he is accepted for training. However, the actual circuit never stays the same for consecutive courses in order to stop potential recruits training specifically. The SBS need all-round fitness and, as with all the training, the instructors love dishing out surprises. The Test is scored on each individual exercise and the total added up. A good start is 550 points while above 700 is very good. Our pass mark is 625 (Marines average 720!).

Guidelines and Training Tips

- If you have passed the Beast after Week 8, you should already be very fit but you should leave 2-3 weeks to get ready for the SBS Challenge.
- Try each exercise on a regular basis to really get to know it. Practise each on its own and in groups of 2-3.
- Buy any necessary equipment – like a pull-up bar.
- If you have a pull-up bar put it in the kitchen doorway. Every time you go through the door do 3 pull-ups. Your strength will increase dramatically.
- Make boxes and lateral jump bar.
- Train 6 days a week with one Complete Rest Day.
- Stick to Active Rest programme (Week 8) but run at least once every week and use that phase to use the route applicable to the test.
- Rest for 2 days before the Test – just stretch and mobilise.

Diet Tips

- Do **NOT** carbo load. People rarely get it right. Just increase your carbohydrate intake throughout the week.
- Power bars are great to snack on, if a little expensive. Eat one 30 minutes before training washed down with a litre of water.
- Stay hydrated – drink at least 2 litres of water a day.
- Have a big bowl of pasta the evening before – but not too late. Give the body time to digest, and get lots of sleep.

- Do **NOT** do the Challenge less than two hours after eating (power bars excepted).
- Eat a high-carb meal about an hour after the test to replenish energy.

Instructions

The circuit is usually carried out in pairs, with one person working and the other counting. Take 2 minutes rest after the run, 1 minute between every other exercise. This is a real killer on the legs but the SBS need strong legs for their work – so be ready to die.

Exercise	Time	Points
3-Mile run	20 minutes for 100 points	add or subtract 3 points for every 15 seconds under or over 20 minutes
Pull-ups	maximum you can do	5 points per pull-up
Sit-ups	2 minutes	1 point per rep
Box jumps	1 minute	10 points per rep
Press-ups*	1 minute maximum	1 point per press-up
Dorsal raises	1 minute	1 point per rep (watch out for cheating – lift your legs and chest off the ground at the same time)
Burpees	1 minute	2 points per rep
Incline sit-ups	1 minute	1 point per rep
Military presses	1 minute	1 point per rep
Lateral jumps	1 minute	1 point per rep

* A partner must be able to put a clenched fist on the floor under your chest for it to qualify as a real press-up.

Box jumps

Place three boxes 1.5 metres apart, they should start at 60 cm (2 ft) high then decrease to 45 cm (18 inches), and 30 cm (12 inches). Two footed take-off, land over each box, then run back to the start.

Military presses

For real SBS selection, this would be replaced by a rope climb. If you have a 6 metre (20 ft) high rope, use it. Climb to maximum; 10 points per climb (no rest between climbs).

Motivation Tips

- Psyche yourself up for the test – mentally you must be prepared.
- Do not worry about points first time out. Just do the circuit. Improvement in your points tally **will** come.
- Get someone to do the Challenge with you or get them to watch, count, and time the exercises to increase your motivation.
- Remember this test is designed to test the fittest soldiers in the world. Keep it in perspective.

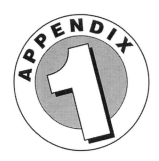

Love Your Feet

Simon Costain is a podiatrist who specialises in the non-surgical management of foot problems and the problems caused by foot malfunction – wonky knees, shin splints and sore Achilles tendons. He runs the renowned Gait and Posture Centre in Harley Street and in 1992 was the podiatrist for the British Olympic Team. Five years ago he was asked by Royal Navy Surgeon Commander Tim Douglas-Riley to help reduce the number of lower limb injuries that the Royal Marines were suffering in training.

Among his recommendations was to replace the concrete surfaces, which they would land on with great impact when exercising, with gravel. Another was to consider changing the standard issue running shoes. 'With all due respect these shoes were fairly cheap and big lads were running in these shoes, which were collapsing,' says Simon. 'I had to impress upon everyone the importance of *preventative* care. People don't look after their feet enough.'

During an average lifetime each foot will walk around the earth between seven and ten times – 250,000 miles. Each day the cumulated weight each foot takes is around 500 tons. Sometimes it's hard to believe that the 26 bones in a foot can take all that pressure.

If one has not been taking regular exercise for a while, it is important to take good care of your feet. Simon believes that many injuries are caused by mechanical factors. If your knee hurts it may be because you have been running on concrete too much. So be aware. 'Your typical injury-prone 30-year-old runner is the single line plodder,' explains Simon. 'If you jog at the same pace, wear the same shoes over the same course day after day, you will be employing the same muscles in the same areas. You are much more likely to injure yourself doing that than if you change your shoes, alternate the surfaces and terrain, and vary your running style and stride length.'

What Shoes?

The key is getting the right shoes. The wrong ones can cause injury. When Robin first started running he bought a pair of cheap trainers, and within two months his knees were aching constantly. They'd be fine out running but within half an hour they were throbbing. When he was in New Zealand writing an article on the England cricket team, he sought advice from the team physiotherapist, Laurie Brown. Laurie didn't look at his knee first but his running shoes. The next day Robin bought a better pair with much more shock absorption. His sore knees went away for two years. Then following a serious Achilles/calf tear he kept getting minor aches and pulls. Eventually he went to see Simon Costain who designed some orthotic soles to minimise the problem. They are still going strong. So are his legs.

A year later during step aerobic sessions Robin started getting twinges inside his kneecap. After a session he would have to sit down for half an hour, while his knees groaned and ground together. The cause was once again his shoes. To save money he was using his wonderful running shoes for step and circuit work. So he bought a pair of Nike Air Trainer Press cross trainers and now he very rarely gets knee twinges.

While doing circuits do not wear running shoes. Modern running shoes are designed purely for running in a straight line – they have tremendous shock absorption properties but the uppers are very light and flimsy. When your foot turns suddenly, it finds no support which puts extra unexpected pressure on the lower leg. If your circuit training involves regular and heavy weight-lifting activity, you should consider a shoe that gives extra ankle support – Robin uses Nike Air Trainer Max.

Invest in a good pair of cross trainers, or tennis or squash shoes. In general the more you pay for a cross trainer the better the shoe. That is not the case with running shoes. Only 15 per cent of running shoes are sold to dedicated runners, the rest are fashion accessories.

If you want to spend a lot on trainers buy two pairs instead – a cross trainer and medium priced running shoe. You can run short distances (3-4 miles) in a good pair of cross trainers but if you're going to be covering greater distances on a regular basis invest in runners too. Don't just buy any old pair. Go to a dedicated running or sports shop where they know what they are talking about. It is best to stick to the well-known brands – you pay a bit more but at least you know they'll help, not hinder, your feet.

If you walk a lot on concrete and tarmac it's worth considering cushioning the impact with insoles. Spencer heel lifts and Sorbathane heel pads both help to reduce excess strain on the heel. Sorbathane do a full insole which may be useful if you are suffering regular pain.

The American company Rockport has a standard street shoe that is as light as a running shoe. The Marathon Brogue has been tested in a Marathon and yet it looks as if it belongs beneath a pinstripe suit. Rockport also do a boot that Robin wishes he'd known about when he was training for the Commando Thirty Miler. Designed using sports technology, it's hard wearing, lightweight, waterproof and comfortable.

Foot Exercises

Simon Costain recommends the following to increase strength in your feet.

1 Ball and the wall

Take off your shoes. Stand on one leg with the other tucked behind. With your right hand gently throw a tennis ball at the wall, catch it with your left hand. Do this for 5 minutes, then swap legs and repeat.

2 Modified Rhomberg test

Stand barefoot on one leg like a stork. Hold both arms out from your body in a T-shape. Close your eyes. Keeping your balance is hard work and strengthens the feet muscles. Swap legs and repeat until you fall over.

Self-foot massage

Sylvia Klein Otkin recommended the following techniques for self-foot massage in 'Massage For Runner' in *Running and Fitness* back in 1983. It works.

1 Sitting on a chair, place one bare foot on the opposite thigh. Rub a bit of massage oil – almond or coconut – on your hand and apply to the foot.

2 Using your thumbs, apply pressure as you work from the bottom of the arch to the top near the big toe. Repeat five times.

3 Make a fist and use the knuckles to move from the heel area to the toes. Repeat five times.

4 Squeeze the fleshy part of the sole together by intermeshing your fingers and squeezing the foot between them.

5 Hold all the toes with one hand and bend them backwards. Hold for 5-10 seconds. Move the toes in the opposite direction. Hold. Repeat this sequence three times.

6 Concentrate on the three useful pressure points on the feet and ankles described below. By working these points, which are usually quite sensitive, you make your legs feel lighter and somewhat tingly.

Pressure point 1 is almost in the centre of the foot. The area is sensitive and slightly hollowed so your thumb should fit well. Using the pad of your thumb apply firm pressure for 30 seconds.

Pressure point 2 is on the inside of the foot just below the bone of the big toe. Use the pad of the thumb and massage in a circular motion for 30 seconds.

Pressure point 3 is located four fingers up from the ankle bone on the inside of the leg. Place your left hand on your right ankle. Using the thumb pad, press in behind the bone next to where your fingers end. Keep massaging until this area feels warm, relaxed and less sensitive.

Coping with Injuries

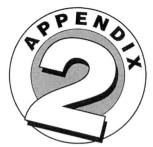

To get maximum gains from exercise an individual needs to work hard and with hard physical activity comes a degree of discomfort. But, unless you are a masochist, pain must not be confused with good results. With an increase in physical fitness you will be able to work harder, and your pain threshold will increase. There's a subtle difference between pushing yourself hard and pushing yourself over the edge.

Muscle soreness is caused by the waste products that build up each time a muscle is worked. The harder you work the muscles, the more these by-products will build up. The most common is lactic acid. Large rises in lactic-acid production also cause muscle stiffness. This can be reduced by a good cool-down, which not only helps return heart rates to pre-exercise levels but also helps dispel waste products.

Anaerobic exercise – eg sprinting – will cause the onset of pain more quickly as your muscles are working at a high rate but with less oxygen, so waste products will build up and with them come pain. Aerobic exercise – eg marathon running – will cause less pain because oxygen is present in large enough quantities to reduce the effects of waste products.

So don't overwork. Listen to your body. Don't carry on regardless if you feel unwell or in pain which doesn't vanish quickly by reducing your activity or resting. Use your common sense. Remember that overexercise is as bad as no exercise. But like death and taxes injuries do happen. The most common form of injuries during Marine recruit training are overuse injuries – specific and non-specific. A specific injury is a stress fracture. General knee pain, aching in the shins, or sore Achilles tendons are non-specific. The majority of injuries are to the lower limbs, followed by back problems and lastly upper limb injuries.

Stress fractures

Stress fractures in Marine training are caused by the constant pounding of heel and sole in boots not designed by an orthopaedic surgeon. A series of small bruises or pressures continues to build up until something gives – a bone in the shin or foot cracks under the pressure. Such injuries are unlikely for anyone following circuit training. However if the pain gradually increases in a local area during exercise, and continues to grow, eventually you will be unable to carry any weight at all. Listen to your body and if it hurts like hell, stop, and consult a doctor. A stress fracture can take six to eight weeks to heal. The only real cure is rest.

Ankles

Going over or turning the ankle is a common injury. If you run on woodland paths, roots or undergrowth will often make you lose your footing and turn over your foot. The more you turn over your ankle the more prone you become to this type of injury. It tends to stretch the ligaments holding the ankle joint in place which makes the joint slack. A bad turn leads to pain in the local area, and there may be swelling, bruising and discoloration. In the worst cases you can't put any weight on the leg.

Rest, Ice, Compression and Elevation (the RICE cure, see page 138) is the best form of treatment, but if this hasn't worked in two days or the symptoms get worse then consult a doctor. Depending on the degree of strain or sprain, try to start exercising the ankle after three days by gently taking the ankle joint through its full range of movement. Follow this by partial weight-bearing exercises such as double-footed heel raises – as the pain decreases start balancing on the injured foot, and then try balancing on one leg with your eyes closed. Then it is time to return to normal activities.

If you are constantly going over on your ankles, place your training shoes on a flat surface at eye level and then look for excessive wear. If they look dodgy get a new pair. Today, you can get shoes which are designed to stop you turning in or turning out. If in doubt get a friend to run with you and to watch you very carefully from the rear when you are getting tired. Weakness shows up the more tired you are.

Knees

The knee joint is a huge joint with a small amount of pivoting, which is prone to injury. It's a complicated mechanism that medical science has not yet been able to replicate artificially, though it has made tremendous advances in the last 20 years. Most knee injuries affect one or more of the ligaments which hold it together.

Most of the knee problems encountered in the Marines are non-specific, complaints about pain in and around the knee joint. These pains could be caused by a sudden increase in physical activity or growing pains. Marines tend to treat them by simply reducing the stress placed through the joint – avoiding long runs, weighted bending and other exercises which induce pain. At the same time they increase exercises to strengthen the quadriceps and hamstrings which will reduce the amount of strain put on the knee.

If you hurt your knee beyond a twinge, you will have pain in and around the injury site, it will swell fairly rapidly after initial injury, there will be a loss of mobility and a reduction in weight-bearing ability. Start treatment with the RICE cure but if symptoms persist or worsen or if swelling is red and hot to the touch consult a doctor. If injury responds to RICE then after two or three days start gentle mobilisation of the joint followed by strengthening of the quads and hamstrings. In all cases with lower limb injuries when you are getting better WALK before you run.

Back problems

In the Marines most back problems occur in the lower back caused by the weight of carrying equipment. The most common cause is poor lifting practice. In civilian life we're not talking just about heavy packs or lifting barbells – we are also called upon to help lift a filing cabinet, a child or even a heavy bag of shopping. When you are lifting *any* weight at all try to ensure that you have a flat lower back and you use your legs to supply the lifting force – *not* the muscles in the lower back.

If something goes, rest first then consult a doctor or physiotherapist. As the symptoms reduce, start gentle mobilising exercises, then gradually build up strength.

Soft tissue injuries

Most soft tissue injuries – aches, tweaks, twinges, turns, sprains and strains – can be avoided with a good warm-up and stretch. However they do occur. If you feel discomfort, pain, a twinge or tightness in a muscle while exercising then STOP. If it appears to be a minor ache rub it and mobilise the joints. If the pain has stopped you can start exercising again, but if the discomfort returns at all STOP IMMEDIATELY.

Analysing injuries

If you get a sudden severe and unexpected pain you should always stop exercise at once. However if after a couple of days' rest you exercise and it comes back again, this indicates that you are doing something wrong. Let's assume you have an insidious pain in the knee that comes on gradually during a sesh. This indicates that some other mechanism is not working properly and the effect is being felt in the knee.

Reduce the exercise routine you are doing but carry on with other variations. Start to analyse your activities, and change them. If you run on roads, run on grass for a while. Consider changing your shoes for a pair that don't allow so much lateral movement, which might have put an extra twist on the knees. Perhaps you have been getting sharp pains in the shins. Go to your local pool and try running in about 4 feet of water. If the pain stops you need more shock absorption in your shoes, so try adding a pair of Sorbathane insoles.

If you get injured, don't just give up and sulk. Try to work out what the problem may be. The more you understand how your own body works the easier it is to push it. But if the pain persists don't be a macho idiot. Seek medical advice. Sometimes not exercising is better for you. Remember most injuries are avoidable. If you warm up correctly and listen to your body then you should remain relatively injury free. If you feel real pain then stop. You might gain macho points for carrying on but if you can't walk for a week you have to ask whether that is a sensible swap.

The best motto is: if in doubt leave it out.

The RICE cure for minor muscular injuries

RICE is the most underrated way of treating minor injuries yourself. It stands for: **R**est, **I**ce, **C**ompression, **E**levation.

Rest Rest the injured limb, or whole body if advised, until the treatment is complete.

Ice Apply an ice pack to the injured area for 10 minutes every hour possible for 48 hours. Don't put ice directly on to the skin (wrap it in a tea towel or similar to prevent skin burns). You can now buy proper ice-pack bandages which are very good.

Compression Bandage the area firmly (but not so tightly as to reduce blood flow) in order to contain the swelling. Use anti-inflammatory drugs from the chemist after consulting your doctor. Continue to use an elastic bandage as long as there is swelling. If it is localised it can be difficult to obtain even compression, so place a piece of soft foam over the area, then put on an elastic bandage. However, if you need a bandage on an injury you really shouldn't be training.

Elevation Elevate the injured limb on a couple of pillows so that the injured area is above the heart. This allows blood to flow towards the heart and reduces the pressure of fluid on the injured area. If you are elevating a foot, make sure the knee is also supported. If the injury persists see a doctor.

When you start training again do so at a lower level. If the injury threatens to be long term wherever possible do not omit to exercise other parts of the body – keeping fit should speed your recovery time. Don't be a fool and try too hard too soon. Further aggravating an injury could mean months not weeks out of action.

Hunter Troop remedial circuits for lower limb injuries

Down at Commando Training Centre in Lympstone, recruits who injure themselves during training too seriously to continue with their original troop become members of Hunter Troop, where they spend as much time as possible getting back into shape before they have any chance of winning their green beret.

As with any injury that affects a joint, you must try to maintain the muscles that operate the joint in order to reduce rehabilitation time. During the early stages it is also important to maintain the mobility and strength of the unaffected joints and muscles. The seriousness of the injury will determine the level of the physical activity you should start with. Always seek medical advice before undertaking any form of exercise.

Just because you have hurt your legs does not mean that you cannot continue to exercise the upper body! Do the following exercises once a day. The number of reps will depend on your physical fitness and the severity of your injury. Remember that pain is an indication of too much work. Listen to your injuries and don't run until you can walk without discomfort.

Early Knees (a term used by the RAF Rehabilitation Centre)

(Inability to bear weight on injured leg and in the early stages of rehabilitation after injury)

In conjunction with these exercises, you could also try cycling on a stationary bike or other non weight-bearing exercise such as swimming or rowing.

STATIC QUAD

Sitting in relaxed position on chair with one leg extended, heel resting on floor, tense front thigh muscles of extended leg and hold for 5 seconds. Swap legs and repeat.

QUAD EXTENSIONS

Sit on chair with back straight and feet flat on floor. Keeping knees together, raise one leg in front, with foot flexed, and hold for 2 seconds. Return leg to floor and repeat. Repeat with other leg.

CALF RAISES

Sit in relaxed position on chair. Holding on to seat of chair, lift one heel off floor. Hold for 2-5 seconds. Lower heel, and repeat. Repeat with other foot.

STRAIGHT LEG RAISING AND CHOPPING

Sit on floor with legs extended and support yourself on hands. Tense front thigh muscles and raise legs about 20-45 cm (8-18 inches) off floor. From here, move legs up and down in scissor-like motion as many times as injury allows.

STATIC HAMSTRING

Lie face down on floor. Raise one leg off floor slightly. Tense buttock muscles of raised leg by pushing leg down to floor. Hold for 5 seconds. Repeat with other leg.

HAMSTRING CURLS

Lie face down with legs extended. Keeping thighs on floor, bend one knee and raise heel towards backside. Hold for a 2 seconds, then return leg to floor and repeat. Repeat with other leg. To increase resistance, place light weights around ankles.

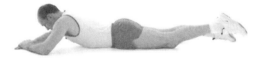

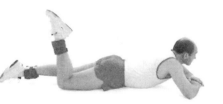

Intermediate Knees

(Partial weight-bearing with a good range of movement)

In conjunction with the following exercises, you could try cycling (on stationary bike), rowing (on machine or boat) or brisk walking (gradually increase pace to a gentle jog) on an absorbent surface.

QUAD EXTENSIONS

As Early Knees, but place light weights around ankles or use an elastic band to increase resistance.

CALF RAISES

Sit on chair with feet flat on floor. Lift heel of one foot off floor while pressing down on knee with hands to increase resistance. Hold for 2-5 seconds. Lower heel to floor, and repeat. Repeat with other foot.

STEP-UPS

Use low bench (approx. 20 cm/8 inches) or use step machine in gym. Lead first with injured leg. Concentrate on working in a pain-free range.

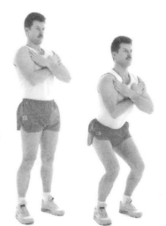

HALF SQUATS

Stand upright with feet shoulder-width apart, hands crossed on chest or holding on to a chair for support. Bend knees and go down into a semi-squat position. Return to starting position and repeat.

FORWARD LUNGES

Perform with control and only lunge as far as injury allows. Hold on to a chair for support if necessary.

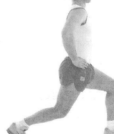

Early Legs

(Inability to bear weight on injured leg)

In conjunction with the following exercises, try cycling on a stationary bike, or other non weight-bearing exercise such as swimming or rowing.

QUAD EXTENSIONS

As Early Knees but place light weights around ankles to increase resistance.

CALF RAISES

As Early Knees.

STATIC QUAD WITH LEG CHOPPING

Sit on chair with back straight and feet flat on floor. Tense front thigh muscles of one leg and extend leg in front, level with other knee. Lower the leg, and repeat with other leg. Continue alternating legs times as many times as injury allows.

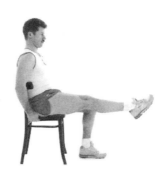

STATIC HAMSTRING WITH LEG CHOPPING

Lie face down on floor with legs extended. Tense buttock muscles of one leg and, keeping leg straight, raise it off floor. Lower the leg to the floor, and repeat with other leg. Continue alternating legs as many times as injury allows.

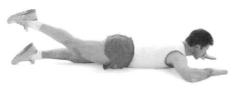

HAMSTRING CURLS

As Early Knees.

ANKLE DORSIFLEXION

Lie on your back with knees bent. Extend injured leg out on the floor, resting calf on a cushion if necessary. Move ankle up and down. Swap legs and repeat.

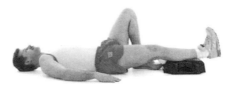

Intermediate Legs

(Partial weight-bearing with a good range of movement)

In conjunction with the following exercises, cycling (on stationary bike), swimming, brisk walking and gentle jogging are also recommended if your injury allows.

QUAD EXTENSIONS

As Early Knees, but place weights or elastic band around ankles to increase resistance.

CALF RAISES

As Intermediate Knees.

STEP-UPS

As Intermediate Knees.

HALF SQUATS

As Intermediate Knees.

FORWARD LUNGES

As Intermediate Knees.

HAMSTRING CURLS

As Early Knees.

TRUNK CURLS

Can also be performed bringing just one knee in towards chest, but make sure you do an equal number of reps with each leg.

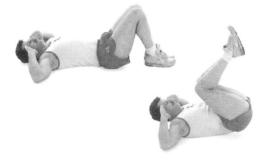

Upper Limbs

Once again the most important parameters are to work the unaffected joints and muscles during the early stages. After two weeks in a plaster cast, even if it is unaffected by the initial injury, the elbow will lose its ability to work throughout its range of movement.

The majority of upper limb injuries are either fractures of the fingers/wrist to soft tissue injuries such as muscle sprains, or they are joint injuries like dislocations. Even if you are in a sling you can exercise other unaffected joints by taking them through their various ranges of movement.

Trunk Injuries

The main area of injury is the back. Millions of working days are lost a year due to back injuries but most can be avoided by correct lifting techniques, good flexibility and strengthening exercises. The extent of your injury will determine the level of exercise you start at.

Hydrotherapy

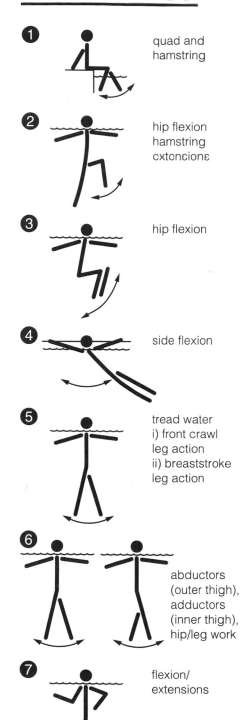

1 quad and hamstring

2 hip flexion hamstring extensions

3 hip flexion

4 side flexion

5 tread water
i) front crawl leg action
ii) breaststroke leg action

6 abductors (outer thigh), adductors (inner thigh), hip/leg work

7 flexion/extensions

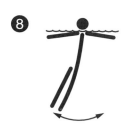

8 trunk swinging

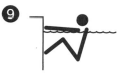

9 passive flexion lower limb

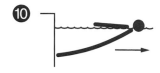

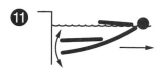

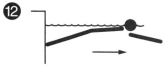

10 push and glide on front and back

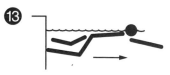

11 push and glide with front crawl or back leg kicks

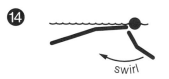

12 push and glide with double leg (dolphin)

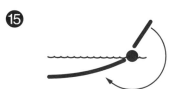

13 push and glide with breast-stroke leg kicks

14 arms only with a float if necessary emphasise the swirl with hands

swirl

15 backstroke, arms only double arm pulls

In the case of serious injuries the best place to exercise can be in a swimming pool as the water supports the body and prevents too much weight bearing. You can carry out an entire circuit in the water. Here is a sequence of 15 suggested exercises. Be sensible about how long you exercise for and if you start to feel pain then STOP.

COPING WITH INJURIES

Exercise Index

When designing your own circuit (see pages 128-9), you can use this index to refer back to the instructions for the key circuit exercises. Remember to use a Whole Body Approach and include a balanced selection of Arm, Trunk and Leg exercises.